Patient participation in palliative care

A Voice for the Voiceless

Edited by

Mrs Barbara Monroe
Chief Executive
St Christopher's Hospice, Sydenham, London, UK

and

Mr David Oliviere
Director of Education and Training
St Christopher's Hospice, Sydenham, London, UK

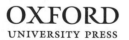

OXFORD
UNIVERSITY PRESS

OXFORD

UNIVERSITY PRESS

Great Clarendon Street, Oxford OX2 6DP

Oxford University Press is a department of the University of Oxford.
It furthers the University's objective of excellence in research, scholarship,
and education by publishing worldwide in

Oxford   New York

Auckland   Bangkok   Buenos Aires   Cape Town   Chennai
Dar es Salaam   Delhi   Hong Kong   Istanbul   Karachi   Kolkata
Kuala Lumpur   Madrid   Melbourne   Mexico City   Mumbai   Nairobi
São Paulo   Shanghai   Taipei   Tokyo   Toronto

Oxford is a registered trade mark of Oxford University Press
in the UK and in certain other countries

Published in the United States by Oxford University Press Inc., New York

A catalogue record for this title is available from the British Library

Library of Congress Cataloging in Publication Data
(Data available)

ISBN 0 19 851581 2

10   9   8   7   6   5   4   3   2   1

Typeset by Cepha Imaging Pvt Ltd, India
Printed in Great Britain
on acid-free paper by Biddles Ltd, Guildford and King's Lynn

WB 310

Patient participation in palliative care

Preface

Developing a creative alliance with the *person* beyond the *patient* is a core tenet of effective palliative care. This book explores the meaning, purposes, value and delivery of person-centered palliative care. In creating St Christopher's Hospice in 1967 and thereby launching the modern hospice movement, Dame Cicely Saunders drew on the strength of the voices of so many who had until then remained voiceless, the dying. As Professor John Hinton (1967) observed at around the same time 'the dissatisfied dead cannot noise abroad the negligence they have experienced'. Saunders' hundreds of meticulously documented tape recordings of patients discussing their individual experiences made sure that this situation did not continue. Paradoxically although many of today's governments themselves now issue demands for user involvement in healthcare, as settings multiply along with their associated experts, treatments and technologies, the need for a better understanding of how to develop active partnerships between service users and professionals has never been greater. This book examines progress thus far and attempts to delineate future challenges.

The book places the modern hospice movement in a context characterized by the need for instant information, a better-informed public more able to criticize and with greater expectations of choice and solutions, a multi-cultural society and a tension between the roles and rights of the traditional specialist expert and the individual user. All of these factors interact within an expectation that users will be involved actively. Part 1 considers the political and philosophical evolution of current developments in user involvement in palliative care, continuing by addressing specific key areas such as quality, education, the role of culture and bereavement care. In Part 2 various professionals give a perspective of how the particular value base, knowledge and practice of their profession attempts to maximize person-centred and user-involved work.

There is sometimes confusion over the use of different terms such as person centred and user involvement. Part of the richness of palliative care is that these concepts are in evolution. We are using person centred to relate to the individual in the holistic model of total care. Being person centred is a dynamic two-way process. Indeed patients and professional staff repeatedly testify to how much they receive from one another. User involvement is concerned with the means of achieving a person-centred service and the meaningful participation and consultation of service users—the people who are the patients, clients and carers of palliative care—in the planning, evolution, evaluation and education of services from their own unique perspective.

Professionals in palliative care settings often somewhat glibly state that the patient is, or should be, at the centre of care. There have been few attempts to examine how to keep them there without professional needs and protocols crowding them out. This book asks how we listen and why we listen. As Relf reminds us in her chapter, listening is not a neutral activity and we need to develop a much more sophisticated understanding of the differing filters of conceptual frameworks that can get in the way of effective dialogue between service user and service deliverer. Having listened we must also seek appropriate ways to act upon what we hear, supporting and promoting the voices that emerge.

Small and Bradburn pursue this theme, exploring how to develop alliances that deal with power imbalances and that ensure that users become not just commentators on services but actively involved in their development and implementation. They examine the best structures to ensure that users can organize to put relevant pressure on healthcare planners. Napier continues this examination by reminding us that very ill people are not sovereign consumers able to pick and choose freely in the market place. Their choices are inevitably limited and they do need the support of experts, particularly since most users of palliative care services are unaware of what would constitute a good service until they actually need it. Gilbert sounds a warning about the dangers of suppressing the shared professional values of healthcare workers, which must remain a fundamental part of what is offered to patients and their families. Speck, Davie and Noble provide a reminder that professionals can be too quick to classify service users as vulnerable and that many of them readily see the personal benefits of participating in research and education, provided explicit conditions of support are met.

Finally, there are of course, the ongoing challenges that palliative care faces in reaching out vigorously to advocate for those excluded from good care; the disenfranchised, disadvantaged and discriminated against. When we are working with patient, family and friendship networks, whose choice matters most? How do we make sure that those with rare conditions or where death comes very quickly, or those who leave no one grieving for them, or who have only professional carers in institutions, also have their voices heard? How do we ensure that our efforts to find representative voices do not diminish important differences in class, gender and ethnicity?

Small remarks that there is 'an impetus for innovation that comes from the memory of things done badly, a perception that things can be done better, an idea of how to achieve this and a picture of what a better system could look like.' The voices of users, patients, carers and professional stakeholders are vital to the process of understanding and achieving shared and relevant quality agendas. The end product of user involvement and person-centred care is to offer the best possible experience in palliative care. As the thoughts of the service users that end this book demonstrate, both done well can enhance energy, choice and the value of individuals everywhere.

We thank all who have contributed to the ongoing debate about the nature of person-centred palliative care and the part user involvement plays within it. In particular, thanks to Jan Stone for her painstaking typing of repeated drafts of the text and to the numerous people with whom we have worked, patients, carers and colleagues, who continue to inspire and challenge us.

Reference

Hinton, J (1967) *Dying*. Penguin, Middlesex, UK.

BM
DO

Contents

List of contributors

Professor Sam H. Ahmedzai
Professor of Palliative Medicine
Sheffield Palliative Care Studies Group, The University of Sheffield

Jane Bradburn
Research and Development Consultant, Cancer Voices
Macmillan Cancer Relief

Fiona Broughton
Palliative care patient

Emma Davie
Bereavement Consultant
Palliative Care Unit, Northern General Hospital, Sheffield

Pam Firth
Head of Family Support
Isabel Hospice, Welwyn Garden City

Dr James Gilbert
Medical Director
Hospiscare, Exeter

John Hunt
Research Fellow
Sheffield Palliative Care Studies Group, The University of Sheffield

Christine Kalus
Consultant Clinical Psychologist
The Rowans, Portsmouth

Professor Alwyn Lishman
Bereaved carer

Barbara Monroe
Chief Executive
St Christopher's Hospice

Lindsey Napier
Senior Lecturer
University of Sydney

Dr Bill Noble
Senior Lecturer
Sheffield Palliative Care Studies Group, The University of Sheffield

Dr Juan M. Núñez Olarte
Associate Professor of Medicine
Hospital General Universitario Gregorio Marañón, Madrid

David Oliviere
Director of Education and Training
St Christopher's Hospice

Dr Marilyn Relf
Bereavement Services Manager
Sir Michael Sobell House, Oxford

Dame Cicely Saunders
Founder/President
St Christopher's Hospice

Professor Neil Small
Professor of Community and Primary Care
University of Bradford

Reverend Peter Speck
Trust Chaplaincy Team Leader
Southampton University Hospitals (NHS) Trust

Mandy Stratford
Patient Services Manager
Arthur Rank House, Cambridge

Part 1

The role of the patient in palliative care

1

A voice for the voiceless

Dame Cicely Saunders

Nurses, social workers, doctors and other professionals hear different questions and comments from patients. As they begin to fear that their illness is not responding to treatment, people will sometimes test staff they know cannot give them answers. These staff can only suggest that the question be put to those who, certainly in the past, may have been seen as guardians of an unpleasant truth. No one *wants* bad news but uncertainty and constantly dashed hopes are often harder to bear. A much admired Ward Sister, referring to a demanding patient, said to her staff one evening 'That man needs to talk' and went to open an exchange which manifestly relieved much overwhelming and previously unaddressed anxiety. This was indeed bold when, during those War years, so little information was given. Because of that restriction, a junior nurse was often treated with an easy camaraderie by patients and who knows how much ease that gave to both parties. Having no responsibility can be frustrating but can also avoid much tension and lead to a relaxed banter. Memories of those pre-antibiotic days when pharmacopeia was limited and when there was nothing to offer but meticulous nursing and the often intimate relationships that developed, are an important part of my own therapeutic journey (Saunders 1996).

Social workers were among the first to keep detailed observations of the inadequate provision available for end-of-life care. One seminal article from Boston was published in the *New England Journal of Medicine* in 1945 (Abrams *et al.* 1945). Four social workers plotted the course of 200 patients and noted a serious gap in communication as well as in service provision. Further studies by social workers illustrated the journeys they shared with their dying patients and their families as they tried to help them discover their own strengths (Saunders 2001).

It was as a Lady Almoner (medical social worker) that I met David Tasma from the Warsaw Ghetto, a patient in the large teaching hospital I was working in during the summer of 1947. He could only be offered palliative surgery and, knowing that he faced a relapse, I kept in touch with him after his discharge and during his admission to another hospital for terminal care some months later. During the following two months I was virtually his only visitor and, in an increasingly deeper relationship, discussed with him the possibility of founding somewhere more suited to his need (he was then a patient on a busy surgical ward of some 60 patients). This need was not only for better symptom control, but also for an opportunity to come to a sense of fulfilment of a solitary life, ending as it was at the age of 40 in a foreign land. Speaking of his legacy to me of £500 he said, 'I will become a window in your Home.' He thus became the founder of the modern hospice and palliative care movement. On another occasion he asked 'for something to comfort me.' I repeated several psalms to him that I knew by heart and then suggested I might read to him. 'No. I only want what is in your mind and in your heart.' He had become an agnostic, he had told me earlier, but added 'I like you too much to say I believe just because I like you.' Before he died, he told his most understanding Ward Sister that he had come back to the faith of his fathers (his grandfather had been a Rabbi). After his death I felt a strong assurance that he had made a quiet journey to peace in the freedom of the spirit.

His phrases, challenging us to openness, to the match of scientific learning with a relationship of person to person and to that essential inner spiritual freedom, have maintained their place as the founding myth of a now worldwide movement. Such principles have been interpreted and practised in very different cultures and resources.

Patients continue to present us with challenges. Three years after the death of David Tasma, I was working in an early unit for patients with far advanced cancer as a volunteer nurse. It was here that I first observed the effectiveness of regular four hourly giving of oral morphine, established there some years previously by the nursing team. Following the advice of Mr Norman Barrett, the thoracic surgeon for whom I was working at the time, I went on, three years later, to read medicine to learn more about pain.

Whilst working at St Joseph's Hospice in East London with the Irish Sisters of Charity, where I spent seven years on an extensive study on *The Nature and Management of Terminal Pain* (Saunders 1967), I began making tape recordings of many of my patients. The following was presented as part of the annual report of the teaching hospital run by the Sisters in Dublin. I was probably the only Protestant on the staff but had their eager co-operation in the introduction of four hourly opiate oral medication. The patient, Mrs H, was interviewed a week after her admission:

> What was the pain like before you came here?

> Well, it was ever so bad. It used to be just like a vice gripping my spine—going like that and would then let go again—and I didn't get my injections regularly—they use to leave me as long as they could and if I asked for them sometimes, they use to say, 'No, wait a bit longer.' They didn't want me to rely on the drugs that were there, you see. They used to try and see how long I could go without an injection ... I used to be pouring with sweat, you know, because of pain ... couldn't speak to anybody I was in such pain ... and I was having crying fits—I mean I haven't cried, I think I've only cried once since I've been here, that's all—well over a week. And I was crying every other day at the other hospital. I was very depressed, ever so depressed; but I'm not at all depressed here, not like I was there.

> Since you've been here and I put you on regular injections, what's the difference?

> Well, the biggest difference is, of course, this feeling so calm. I don't get worked up, I don't get upset, I don't cry, I don't get very, very depressed—because I was getting awfully depressed, you know, really black thoughts were going through me mind, and no matter how kind people were, and people were ever so kind, nothing would console me you see. But since I've been here I feel more hopeful as well. I feel that I'm getting better and I'm going to go home. Whereas there I didn't, you see. And no-one would tell me that I was either. I kept asking various people, and nobody would give me a clear answer. But since I've been here, I don't feel that desperate need to ask 'Am I going to get better, am I ... ' I mean, I want to know.

> But you don't feel that desperation?

> No, I don't feel that hopelessness.

A much shorter recording was used as part of a Good Cause Appeal on BBC Radio in 1964. Mrs M said:

> Before I came here the pain was so bad that if anyone came into the room I would say, 'Please don't touch me, please don't come near me.' But now it seems as if something has come between me and the pain, it feels like a nice thing wrapped round me.

That same year, I quoted in an article in the *Nursing Times* (Saunders 1964) the answer to the simple question, 'Tell me about your pain.' Mrs T had said,

> Well doctor, the pain began in my back but now it seems that all of me is wrong.

She gave a description of several symptoms and then went on to say,

> My husband and son were marvellous but they were at work and they would have had to stay off work and lose their money. I could have cried for the pills and injections but I knew I mustn't. Everything seemed to be against me and nobody seemed to understand.

She then paused before she said,

> But it is so wonderful to begin to feel safe again.

As I wrote then and many times since, what was being talked about was 'total pain'—'all of me is wrong'. Without any further questioning she had talked of her mental as well as her physical distress, of her social problems and of her spiritual need for security. Then, as now, I know that listening to a patient's own tale of their troubles can be therapeutic in itself. As another patient said, 'It seemed the pain went with me talking.'

One exchange with a particularly well known patient has been used many times in discussions and lectures about the responsibility of giving bad news. Mr A.M. asked directly, 'Am I going to die?'. I replied equally directly with a simple 'Yes' because anything other than such honesty would have been an insult to his dignity. 'Was it hard for you to tell me that?' he asked. When I replied, 'Well, yes, it was' he said, 'Thank you, it is hard to be told but it is hard to tell too. Thank you'. Such conversations should be hard. We should recognize that we are committing our patient to an exacting journey and either to accompanying him ourselves or making sure that other support is available.

Such stories, accompanied by the many photographs I took, were presented in many lectures alongside the increasing volume of statistics showing the lack of tolerance and drug dependence that the regime and the whole hospice milieu was achieving. There were 900 records analysed when this was part of a *Royal Society of Medicine Symposium* (Saunders 1963). I remember a physician remarking then, 'I always thought regular giving worked but didn't know why.' Patients' voices had provided the answer.

Enabling professionals and grant-giving charities to hear these powerful statements led to the opening of the first modern research and teaching hospice, St Christopher's, in 1967. By then, however, the 'movement' (still unnamed) had made considerable progress (Clark 1998). Other patients and frustrated, often despairing, staff had begun to join a mounting interest in a fresh look at end-of-life care. Systematic studies in the 1950s gave necessary breadth to the detailed stories of St Joseph's 1100 patients (Saunders 1967).

From the beginning, St Christopher's had a small number of long-stay patients. Gradually these beds became specialized in the care of patients with motor neurone disease. One such patient, looking at another who was more disabled, said to me 'If I ever get like that man I shall want to do something to myself.' But when he, too, reached that place he said, 'I can't see round the next bend but I know it will be all right.' He went on to suggest a title for a lecture to me. 'This is a "bringing together illness" patient with staff, patient with family.' I asked 'Do you always see it as that?' 'Yes' he replied, with his Police Sergeant look, 'and I'm a trained observer.'

Another patient with motor neurone disease, a former medical secretary, wrote to her brother not long before her death on being the wounded Jew in the parable of the good samaritan instead of the good samaritan himself. These are to me powerful answers to the desperate dependence of increasing paralysis, which people discover if they have supportive care.

Also, of course, only patients themselves can teach us of a patient's own responsibilities. Paula, a still glamorous blond, said to a nurse 'I try not to moan, I just don't want people to remember me as a nasty person.' On her last night, after months of keeping her own counsel on such matters, she suddenly began talking to her night nurse about any life beyond death and asked her what she believed. The nurse was able to say something very simple. Paula replied, 'I can't say I believe now, not like that, but would it be all right if I just said that I hoped?' When she said goodbye to the nurse in the morning, she took off the false eyelashes she wore day and night— 'You can put those away, I won't need them any more.' It was as if she was saying, 'Well, I'm me and it's all right.'

Mr T H wrote an article entitled 'Patiently speaking' for the *Nursing Times* (Holden 1980) with the use of one of the early communicators, a Possum apparatus. In it he gives many hints to those who care for patients with motor neurone and other severely disabling diseases:

> It seems illogical that the only people in hospital who have no training for the occupation are the patients. Would it not make sense to accept that anyone landed in a new and strange environment needs some sort of instruction to help him to fit in and take advantage of the enormous wealth of kindness, generosity and good will, readily given by all staff?

> What the patient has to understand is that although these are rather special people they are people with normal human feelings and responses. They do a very demanding job, work lousy hours for scandalous wages and have their share of trials and tribulations in their private lives. All patients are grateful for the care they get but many do not realise how much their own behaviour can contribute to their and everyone's well-being.

When I suggest that patients could be taught I do not envisage anything overt but judicious, friendly chats could achieve a great deal. Every patient has the right to know the what, why and wherefore about everything from normal routine to his personal treatment and condition. No patient has the right to be constantly complaining, ill mannered, discourteous, jealous, selfish, thoughtless, all the petty things which make *us* so unattractive and will be counter-productive in our relationships with staff, relatives and everyone else. The basic lesson is simple, the greatest act of self-interest is to be as unselfish as possible.

Little needs to be added to these voices, which echo in my memory and which have inspired so many people around the world to listen in their turn. The patients are the founders of the now accepted development of the specialty of palliative medicine.

References

Abrams R, Jameson G, Poehlman M, and Snyder S (1945) Terminal care in cancer. *New England Journal of Medicine*, 232 (25), 726–7.

Clark D (1988) Originating a movement: Cicely Saunders and the development of St. Christopher's Hospice, 1957–1967. *Mortality*, 3 (1), 43–63.

Holden T (1980) Patiently speaking. *Nursing Times.* June 12, pp. 1035–6.

Saunders C (1963) The treatment of intractable pain in advanced cancer. *Proceedings of the Royal Society of Medicine*, 56 (3), 195–7.

Saunders C (1964) Care of patients suffering from terminal illness at St. Joseph's Hospice, Hackney, London. *Nursing Mirror*, February 14, pp. vii–x.

Saunders C (1967) *The Management of Terminal Illness*. Hospital Medicine Publications, London.

Saunders C (1996) Into the valley of the shadow of death—a personal therapeutic journey. *British Medical Journal,* 313, 1599–1601.

Saunders C (2001) Social work and palliative care—the early history. *British Journal of Social Work*, 31, 791–9.

2

The changing National Health Service, user involvement and palliative care

Neil Small

Introduction

From its inception in 1948 the National Health Service (NHS) has undergone major restructurings at regular intervals. It has also seen changes in its operational rationale and in the cultural context it operates within. Its scope for action has changed as have the expectations accepted as legitimate by politicians, planners, service providers, patients and the general public. One recent change has seen the elevation of public and patient involvement to a new prominence.

The modern hospice movement and specialist palliative care has grown up in the UK both alongside and inside the NHS. Even when developments occurred outside the NHS there was always a clear recognition of the need to, as Dame Cicely Saunders said, stay outside, 'so that attitudes and knowledge could move back in' (Saunders, quoted in Taylor 1983). The hospice movement's origins in the late 1940s coincided with the formal establishment of the NHS (Clark 1998). Its institutional birth in 1967 occurred at a time when much innovation in health care was taking place outside and inside the NHS. The development of palliative medicine (formally recognized in 1987) occurred in the context of a more widespread shift towards medical specialism. The proliferation of services in the 1980s occurred at a time when the NHS was expanding but also when it was beginning to recognize that the perennial concerns of escalating costs and of managing services required drastic change (Department of Health 1989; Clark *et al.* 1995).

Throughout its history public involvement has always figured high in hospice thinking. This has been most obviously manifest in the local activism that set up individual hospices and in the need to maintain local support for the finance to allow a hospice to continue. As well as this dimension of public participation the voices of service users can be heard right at the heart of modern hospice development. Dame Cicely Saunders, speaking of her many conversations with David Tasma in Archway Hospital in 1948, reports that, 'it was while we were talking together that the idea [came] of somewhere that would have helped him more ... but the most important thing for him was to find someone who would listen' (quoted in Small 2000). Throughout its subsequent development those in the hospice movement have argued that it, 'grew by listening' (Saunders 1998).

The guiding philosophy of the NHS in its early years combined a belief in the necessity of state intervention to achieve equality and efficiency in health care provision with the idea that the NHS would offer a template for a better sort of society. This represented a coming together of the wartime Beveridge Plan and the vision of the NHS's first Minister of Health, Aneurin Bevan and his supporters (Foot 1975; Webster 1998). Bevan's inspired credo that, 'It is no answer to say that things are better than they were ... the lot of the ordinary man and woman is much worse than it need be' produced the conviction that the space for action was created by the gap between, 'a knowledge of the possible, as contrasted with the actual' (Bevan 1952). Such an approach inspires the sort of restless energy that shifts a sense of discontent into an idea and an idea into a movement.

It was the same for hospice. One influential figure in the UK hospice movement sums this up when he says 'I think the original hospice world promoted itself as a response, as indeed it was to some extent, a response to public demand, to need, to things that were wrong. This was a protest movement, but it was a look at things and saying, "God, things could be better, you know we have got a little section of people here at the most painful, critical, heart breaking time of their lives, and they are being badly looked after, what are we going to do about this thing?" '(quoted in Small 2000).

But that was then, what of now? The election of a Labour Government in May 1997 was followed by a White Paper heralding *The New NHS: Modern, Dependable* (Department of Health 1997*a*) and then *A First Class Service: Quality in the New NHS* (Department of Health 1998*a*). Is what is new about this NHS a sense that restless energy and an aspirational ethic has been replaced by a concern with the detail of service delivery and the minutiae of measuring performance? If we forget why we are doing something does this risk elevating the 'how' to undue prominence, so that we watch our step rather than look at the stars? Or have the times changed so much that the reformist language of the past is no longer relevant? Do we have to reframe the NHS using the constructs of a prevalent consumer culture?[1] A *Guardian* editorial (8 January 2000) argued that these 1997 reforms needed more time to achieve the 'cultural change required in the NHS to provide a service equivalent in accessibility, convenience, reliability and quality to other services available in consumer culture ... It has to be resolved or the middle classes will abandon the NHS.'

While there has been some concern about the sustainability of charitable support for hospice, the more substantial areas of concern have been about the implications of transformation within hospice and about the growth of specialist palliative care. Has an initial reformist agenda been overtaken by a concern with effective management? If the answer is yes, then what is gained and lost in this transition? James and Field (1992) explored the 'routinization of hospice'. James (1994) also spoke of a maturing of the hospice movement as it shifted 'from vision to system'. Hospice always had to fight critics, initially it had to struggle to simply establish itself. Now there are some who have asked if hospices have fulfilled their purpose—that is drawing attention to earlier inadequacies in care of the dying, offering a base for the development of expertise in home care and in nursing skills and acting as a base from which palliative medicine could grow as a speciality (Douglas 1992). More recently a lively debate followed the suggestion that palliative medicine is not best advanced via specialism (Fordham *et al.* 1998; Higginson 1998). Further, the availability of specialist services has provoked scrutiny. How can hospice and specialist palliative care tackle a perception that palliative care operates in a 'comfort zone' and that there are large numbers of 'the disadvantaged dying', those who are too

---

1. In a presentation to the Palliative Care Congress at the University of Warwick in March 2000 I considered how far both the NHS and palliative care are best characterized as seeking to preserve an established ideal or how far they are concerned with a pursuit of the new. I used the device of contrasting the films, *Star Wars* (with its harnessing of 'the force') and *Star Trek* (with the mission of its Starship *The Enterprise* 'to seek out new worlds, to boldly go'). I argued that you could have ideals and innovation but that you needed to judge the latter against the standards of the former and not just assume that the new and the modern were desirable. (For how science fiction film gives an insight into the nature of our modern/postmodern times see Barrett and Barrett 2001.)

old or have the 'wrong' disease, who are not offered this care (Addington-Hall 1999).

Perhaps though only superficials have changed in both the NHS and in palliative care. As the Prime Minister said, 'The values of the NHS are every bit as relevant today as they were 50 years ago. But they have to be applied in a different way for a different age' (Tony Blair in the House of Commons 22, March 2000). In relation to hospice the experience of end-of-life care is, of course, always new for the person receiving that care. They are not likely to be aware of recent debates about the guiding approach to care. Their wants, and the wants of palliative care providers, remain simple and constant: effective control of all those aspects of pain that exist as the end of life approaches and care in a setting the patient would choose, delivered with a sensitivity to the family and social network and in a way that the patient feels they can shape and that reflects their individual needs. To this we can add that their altruism might be reflected in a wish that the sorts of care they receive, if they value it, be available to all who could benefit.

In this scene-setting chapter I will consider what has changed and what stays the same in the NHS. What does the new NHS looks like? Since 1997 there have been a number of crucial developments and I will itemize these. The development of consumerist rhetoric predates the election of the Blair administration and has continued and been, in part, transmuted into a user involvement/public participation approach. I will highlight key features of this progression. I will then consider how changing times and policy initiatives impact on palliative care and specifically will consider how user involvement developed here. The user involvement agenda has gone through a number of stages and these effectively replicate the changing structures and priorities of the NHS rather than reflect user wishes or a judgement about what most advantages involvement. In effect the shape of user involvement has been consequent upon the prevalent ethos of the health service. I will then conclude with a consideration of whether, on balance, the new NHS constitutes an opportunity or a threat for the capacity of palliative care to maximize its achievements and overcome its challenges.

The shape of the new and changing National Health Service

The White Paper *The New NHS: Modern, Dependable* (Department of Health 1997a) established new organizations, planning mechanisms, procedures and priorities. In practice these innovations were often rediscoveries of previous practice or elevations of existing work to a new prominence.

But what appeared to be if not new then rediscovered, was the need to plan—to have priorities and a vision of how one might go about achieving them. This commitment was underlined in *The NHS Plan* (Department of Health 2000a) and in *The NHS Cancer Plan* (Department of Health 2000b).

New organizations included primary care groups (PCGs) and then primary care trusts (PCTs). These would commission as well as deliver services. New ways of accessing health services would include NHS Direct, walk-in and healthy living centres. Two new national organizations were established: the National Institute for Clinical Excellence (NICE) to set standards and approve treatments and the Commission for Health Improvement to act as an inspection service. New ways of planning services included the establishment of health improvement programmes (HIMPs) and health action zones. Both include health and local government planning together. National service frameworks (NSFs) would be established via a rolling programme setting priorities, procedures, targets and standards in one area after another. At a local level clinical governance was to be made more widespread and systemized. New sorts of contracts in primary care would be introduced, the personal medical service contract and salaried doctor services would gradually replace existing general medical services contracts.

At the heart of the new NHS was to be a service that was primary care led. But it was to be a different sort of primary care. There was a shift from an idea of managerialism drawn from business to one that looked to peer pressure to get compliance from professionals. Different governance and a greater emphasis on public accountability means that primary care organizations have to look upwards to the structures of the NHS via national frameworks and targets and via accountability agreements with new strategic health authorities, outwards to local communities, within to their colleagues via contracts and clinical governance and sideways to their patients.

Almost all of the recent NHS changes will have relevance for palliative care. For example commissioning from primary care trusts will involve these new organizations having to decide how much palliative care is needed, what should be provided 'in house' by their own staff and what needs to be commissioned from others. Much of the responsibility for delivering palliative care will remain within primary care. Higginson (1998) identified that in an average general practice with 2500 people, in each year, seven will die of cancer and seventeen from non-cancer conditions like circulatory, respiratory and neurological disorders where there may be a need for palliative care. In the last year of life 90% of care is delivered at home.

The new NHS reconfigures avenues of accountability and generates new points of intersection at which decisions are made. Resource allocation both nationally, in districts and within PCTs will be driven by new structures and processes: the NSFs, NICE guidelines, the structure of the HIMP, local trust priorities and the establishment of clinical governance guidelines. Palliative care needs to have a presence at each of these influential points.

The post 1997 NHS has, even in its short history, been subject to significant shifts of emphasis. In March 2000 the Prime Minister identified to Parliament challenges he felt faced the NHS. There was to be a heightened concern to address major areas of premature mortality in the UK. Heart disease and cancer were to be given special prominence. The shift of emphasis highlights two crucial issues in seeking to understand health policy. First, how difficult it is to set up and keep long-term plans in highly visible and politically volatile public services (see Small 1989). Second, it identifies the various components that need to be in place before things change: data, stories, politics and context.[2] The first two produce pressure, the third decides if the pressure is bearable, the fourth decides the shape of response to that pressure. Rarely is just one of these in evidence, often many of them are. Figure 2.1 provides an example as we look at the shift in policy so that heart disease and cancer would be prioritized.

Another major change since the 1997 White Paper was heralded in the July 2001 Department of Health consultation document *Shifting the Balance of Power* (Department of Health 2001a). This proposed a change in the roles and responsibilities of statutory NHS organizations and their relationship to the Department of Health.

The change was designed to foster networks that work across boundaries between organizations. The intention was to give people the ability to innovate in ways that their professional practice suggested to them and to allow them to do this with other people who could help achieve the same

---

2. While Ministers seek detailed background material from their advisors they are also eager for 'the story', which can help them crystallize why this issue needs to be pursued or that change made. Much policy is narrative led and it is a mistake to think that it is largely the accumulation of evidence in the form of hard data that leads to change. Reading almost any political autobiography can confirm this. The importance of the narrative is also evident in hospice and palliative care development—the personal experience of loss often acting as the catalyst for innovation, the story of when things go wrong, or how successful things have been, helping galvanize support. This is the sort of evidence that inspires action.

Heart disease:
Data: figures showed that 500 patients had been waiting more than a year for by-pass surgery. Each year a similar number died while waiting for surgery.
Story: Ian Weir, a constituent and friend of Alan Milburn MP the Secretary of State for Health, died the day before seeing a consultant about a triple by-pass operation. He had been waiting 7 months for his appointment.

Cancer:
Data: the UK and Denmark had the lowest survival rates in Europe. The UK's record on breast cancer was particularly bad. Professor Gordon McVie of the Cancer Research Campaign argued that with the same resources organized differently (that is, more equally across the population) 25 000 lives a year would be saved.
Story: Mavis Skeet, because of a shortage of beds, had her cancer operation cancelled four times before her doctors declared her condition inoperable.

Politics: A decision to focus resources on heart disease and cancer implies a redistribution within health policy towards conditions of greater severity or life threat.
Context: This change means, in effect, a social redistribution of resources towards the lower social classes. Five times more working class people die of lung cancer and three times as many from heart disease when compared with middle class people.

Fig. 2.1 Influences on policy change.

goals, even if they were in different organizations. This is a change that ought to be supportive of palliative care which characteristically operates via multi-professional networks and across organizational and geographic boundaries.

Contradictions in the participation ethos of the new National Health Service

It is not surprising that there are aspects of the new NHS that are potentially in a relationship of some tension. How far this is creative as opposed to destructive is, as yet, unclear. An emphasis on the importance of involvement by patients and by the public can be in itself a source of tension. A rational assessment of self-interest may mean that one's concerns when one becomes a patient change from those one had as a member of a local community. Similarly for those delivering services, say from inside PCTs, there are tensions between a responsibility to promote the health of one's population—a utilitarian view that sees the need to put an overall population benefit first—with the long-standing Hippocratic approach of putting the individual patient's needs first and foremost.

There is a tension between consumerism, demand-led services and strategic planning, including tackling health inequalities. There is also a tension between consumerism and evidence-based medicine, planning based on best standards of care. It may also be that a patient has to trade off one desired aspect of service for another, for example quick access to any available GP or continuity of care through seeing the same GP at each visit.

There is a tension between local autonomy, for example PCTs commissioning and local HIMPs, and nationally led, top-down, priority and standard setting. This tension impacts on the scope for manoeuvre patients have at local level to effect any meaningful change. For example, *The NHS Cancer Plan* (Department of Health 2000*b*) sets the parameters for the delivery, prioritization and monitoring of cancer services. Cancer networks will cover about 34 PCTs and there will be cancer services collaboratives, which constitute new ways of gathering and implementing evidence and new practice. In the context of these wide-ranging and large-scale innovations the plan also says, in a brief section, 'At a local level cancer networks will be expected to take account of the views of patients and carers when planning services.' In practice this has developed quickly into the idea not of user groups, but of partnership groups which include patients.

Challenges for the future include having to decide how to regulate complex networks and multi-agency team approaches. If we rely on professional self-regulation then in any one area of care or in an individual's health journey there might be many different professions working in different ways. We need to think about how clinical governance and user involvement can encompass care delivered across networks.

User involvement: before and after the 'new National Health Service'

The 1997 White Paper gave a low prominence to the contribution of service users. Rather, it highlighted what was seen as a more pressing agenda, a concern to address public legitimacy and low staff morale. The new NHS was to engage in greater public participation and give health professionals a more enhanced role. In consequence user voices were squeezed out, indeed health professionals were given more authority to define users' needs and there was a tendency to conflate user involvement and public participation (Rhodes and Nocon 1998).

In the years between the introduction of *Working for Patients* (Department of Health 1989) and the 1997 reforms, issues of user involvement had periodically been raised. There had been moves via the *Patients' Charter* (Department of Health 1991) to set out rights and basic service standards for patients. *Local Voices* (Department of Health 1992) indicated how health commissioners could involve local communities in the purchasing process. Consistent with the market approach then prevalent, the approach to user involvement had been a consumerist one (see Croft and Beresford 1990, 1992). 'Choice' was seen as a tool to improve efficiency, effectiveness and economy in service provision. The analogy looked to was retailing—consumers/users will go where they get what they want and not to places that give poor service or bad-quality care. There were a number of short-comings in this scenario: the absence of real choice because of the lack of alternatives; a lack of information about opportunities or transparency about performance; and a sense that this was deficit involvement—that it was about making the not very good a little better. Such an approach, even at its best, can only make an impact on details of what was already in place. It is also reactive, doing something after a problem has been encountered, and individualized, in that is seeks to respond to one person's problem as if it exists in isolation. This was the era when political discourse included the Thatcherite statement that 'there was no such thing as society'.

This approach can be contrasted with a 'politics of empowerment' where the aim is for users to control their own experience of care via having a direct say in what is offered. This is a constructive involvement, engaging with what should be provided. It is essentially collective and proactive. But it is an approach that is problematic in palliative care. For most of us palliative care is a discovered not a conceptualized need. That is, we do not know what would constitute a good service for us until we need it. At that point it is pos-sible that we would have problems in working with others and working for future change, not least because of the demands our illness may place on everyday life (Small and Rhodes 2000). Additional specific challenges for user involvement in palliative care also include the complication of its being a holistic service that offers support to the patient and their family, in a variety of settings including their own home, day care and residential settings. People have a range of needs and severity of symptoms that change as their illness progresses (Oliviere 2001). Who is the user, when are they best involved and how can they contribute across the spectrum of services offered?

User involvement can also detract from a rights-based agenda (Forbes and Sashidharan 1997). Perhaps paradoxically it can be used to help per-petuate existing power structures. If we can claim that users are involved we can profess a legitimacy for what is in place that inhibits opposition. Definitions of need can be limited to the narrow realm of just marginally adding to or taking away from those needs that are already met to some degree. It also excludes those who have been denied or cannot obtain a serv-ice (Osborn 1992). There is a danger that using 'user' as a concept imposes too much uniformity, minimizing differences in class, gender and ethnicity

(Croft and Beresford 1992). The dimension of ethnicity is important not just in terms of practical involvement but in the more fundamental stance people from different ethnic groups might take to issues like autonomy, disclosure, the role of the family and the understanding of suffering (see Field *et al.* 1997). The danger of too easy generalization is compounded when users and carers, who may have very different priorities, are merged into some hybrid 'usercarer' and it is even more marked if user and public involvement are assumed to be synonymous.

These concerns about user involvement are offered not to seek to question its place on the policy agenda, but to offer a benchmark against which initiatives should be judged. The challenge is to be imaginative and get past practical and conceptual problems (the literature on user involvement in general and user involvement in palliative care has been reviewed in Small and Rhodes 2000 and that on user involvement in cancer has been explored in Gott *et al.* 2000, 2002).

Since the 1997 advent of the 'new' NHS, the consumerist model of user involvement has been modified. Consistent with a service that emphasizes a more corporate structure and an evaluative ethos, we have seen policy documents from the Cabinet Office (1998, 1999) and NHS Executive (1999) that have invited wide-ranging considerations of public and user involvement. There has been a continuing concern with the proper place for patient and public participation in the evaluation of health services (Department of Health 2000*a,b*). User involvement in research is being considered (Department of Health 1998*b*) and there are publications highlighting examples of best practice (Department of Health 1997*b*). A discussion document *Involving Patients and the Public in Healthcare* (Department of Health 2001*b*) proposes patients' forums and the establishment of 'Voice'—an independent national body that will serve as a commission for public and patient involvement.

Shifting the Balance of Power (Department of Health 2001*a*) also heralds yet another change in direction when it recognizes that user involvement is not just dependent on having appropriate policies and structures but requires a cultural shift within the health service. It is 'about putting patients and staff absolutely at the heart of the NHS. It does so by giving greater authority and decision making power to patients and frontline staff and underpinning this with changes in organisational roles and relationships.' The specific areas discussed include giving patients more choice and more information, introducing national standards, improving patient safety and creating new partnerships (a necessary feature of a focus on networks). The document 'sets out the framework and principles for those changes' but, in line with its own philosophy, it leaves the practical arrangements, the how, when and where of working arrangements and service delivery 'to be decided locally.'

Innovations continue: national listening exercises, proposals for patients' forums and advice and liaison services in trusts, complaints advocacy services and moves to devise new performance ratings that include patient satisfaction as well as other service outcomes (Department of Health 2001a).

As the NHS ethos and organizational structures have changed so too have the dominant forms of user involvement. We encounter an essentially paternalist service before 1989, then a consumerist approach, which transmutes into a more managerial/corporatist model in the 'New NHS'. *Shifting the Balance of Power* (Department of Health 2001a) then heralds another shift of emphasis into a network-based approach.

The promises and challenges of palliative medicine

We have considered the similarities in the founding principles of the NHS and of hospice care. The shift towards the internal market after 1989 offered challenges and opportunities for hospice and for palliative care. A prioritization of governance, manifest in a concern to pursue and promote evidence, standards and quality has been evident in both the NHS and palliative care in recent years. We have also seen how new configurations in terms of NHS structures generate different points of intersection and different avenues for seeking influence. Pressing issues for palliative care include devising ways of maximizing promise and overcoming challenges (see Fig. 2.2) in this changing context.

Products of the past, custodians of the present, architects of the future

In this chapter I have offered a review of recent changes in the NHS. These changes provide the context for future thoughts about the place of palliative care and about the shape of user involvement. I have suggested that the new NHS means palliative care has to refocus in terms of where it looks for support. Overall the changes offer positive opportunities for palliative care to face its challenges and build on its promises.

Different models of user involvement have developed as the NHS has changed. Users need to ensure they are organizing and putting pressure

---

Promises
- Symptom control to all patients
- To empower other professionals in their management of dying patients
- To recognize and support the skills of general practitioners
- To provide an alternative to fast-paced, thoughtlessly invasive, acute, hospital-style medicine

---

Challenges
- Difficult symptoms
- Moving beyond cancer
- Developing new models of care
- Addressing social exclusion in palliative care
- Developing further user and public involvement
- Furthering the multi-disciplinary team and its members
- Looking to public education
- Developing creative interaction with primary care commissioners
- Consideration of efficacy, equity and value
- Identifying what specialist care can do
- Supporting non-specialists to provide the best service they can

---

Fig. 2.2 Promises and challenges for palliative care.

in a way that maximizes their chances to be influential. For example, it is not advantageous to keep pursuing a consumerist approach when the place decisions are made is in networks. What is needed are innovative projects that test out the scope for change and the limits of the possible across the range of contemporary palliative care.

Like all institutions, the National Health Service in general and palliative care in particular, exist within a complex relationship of what has been done in the past, what can be done in the present and what might be achieved in the future. They encompass forces designed to preserve what is already in place as well as others wanting to move agendas forward. The impetus for change can sometimes be a conservative one—change to protect the organization or to counter forces existing elsewhere within, or outside, the system. But there is also an impetus for innovation that comes from a memory of things done badly, a perception that things can be better, an idea of how to achieve this and a picture of what a better system would look like. The user involvement project is, fundamentally, about how to reconcile the existence of institutional and professional agendas built up out of this longitudinal engagement with service planning and delivery and an agenda built out of the subjective, embodied experience of being ill or caring for someone who is ill. It is an area of activity where different world views exist. It sees the interplay of the utilitarian and future-oriented planners and the needs-and-rights-based concern with the here and now of service users. But these worlds are not hermetically sealed—planners know of the importance of the individual and of the need to get things right for them and users know that one has to make compromises in an area where many have to work together. User involvement will progress if the resulting scope for alliances is developed. The inherent social power of the institutions and professions means that it is incumbent on them to move to meet the user on grounds each can feel is common.

References

Addington-Hall, J. (1999). *Help the Hospices.* National Council for Hospices and Specialist Palliative Care Conference. November.

Barrett, M., Barrett, D. (2001). *Star Trek: The Human Frontier.* Cambridge, Polity Press.

Bevan, A. (1952). *In Place of Fear.* London, Heinemann.

Cabinet Office (1998). *How to Consult your Users.* London, Service First Unit.

Cabinet Office (1999). *Involving Users. Improving the Delivery of Healthcare.* London, National Consumer Council, Consumer Congress and Service First Unit.

Clark, D. (1998). Originating a movement: Cicely Saunders and the development of St Christopher's Hospice. *Mortality,* 3: 43–63.

Clark, D., Small, N., Malson, H. (1995). Hospices to fortune. *Health Service Journal,* 105: 23 November, 30–1.

Croft, S., Beresford, P. (1990). A sea change. *Community Care,* 4 October, 30–1.

Croft, S., Beresford, P. (1992). The politics of participation. *Critical Social Policy,* 35: 20–44.

Department of Health (1989). *Working for Patients.* London, HMSO.

Department of Health (1991). *The Patients' Charter.* London, HMSO.

Department of Health (1992). *Local Voices: the Views of People in Purchasing.* London, NHS Management Executive.

Department of Health (1997a). *The New NHS: Modern, Dependable.* London, Department of Health.

Department of Health (1997b). *Involving Patients: Examples of Good Practice.* London, Department of Health.

Department of Health (1998a). *A First Class Service: Quality in the New NHS.* London, Health Service Circular 113.

Department of Health (1998b). *Research: What's in it for me?* Report from the Standing Advisory Group on Consumer Involvement in NHS Research. London, Department of Health.

Department of Health (2000a). *The NHS Plan.* Leeds, Department of Health.

Department of Health (2000b). *The NHS Cancer Plan: A Plan for Investment, a Plan for Reform.* Leeds, Department of Health.

Department of Health (2001a). *Shifting the Balance of Power.* London, Department of Health.

Department of Health (2001b). *Involving Patients and the Public in Healthcare.* Discussion Document. Leeds, Department of Health.

Douglas, C. (1992). For all the saints. *British Medical Journal,* 303: 579.

Field, D., Hockey, J., Small, N. (1997). *Death, Gender and Ethnicity.* London, Routledge.

Foot, M. (1975). *Aneurin Bevan.* St Albans, Paladin.

Forbes, J., Sashidharan, P. (1997). User involvement in services—incorporation or challenge? *British Journal of Social Work,* 27: 481–98.

Fordham S., Dowrick, C., May, C. (1998). Palliative medicine: is it a really specialist territory? *Journal of the Royal Society of Medicine,* 91: 568–72.

Gott, M., Stevens, T., Small, N., Hjelmeland Ahmedzai, S. (2000). *User Involvement in Cancer Care.* Bristol, Policy Press.

Gott, M., Stevens, T., Small, N., Hjelmeland Ahmedzai, S. (2002). *British Journal of Clinical Governance,* 7.2: 81–5.

Higginson, I. (1998). Who needs palliative care? Editorial. *Journal of the Royal Society of Medicine,* 91: 563–4.

James, N. (1994). From vision to system: the maturing of the hospice movement. In Lee, R., Morgan, D. (eds). *Death Rites. Law and Ethics at the End of Life.* London, Routledge, pp. 102–30.

James, N., Field, D. (1992). The routinization of hospice: charisma and bureaucratization. *Social Science and Medicine,* 34: 1363–75.

NHS Executive (1999). *Patient and Public Involvement in the New NHS.* London, Stationery Office.

Oliviere, D. (2001). User involvement in palliative care services. *European Journal of Palliative Care,* 8: 238–41.

Osborn, A. (1992). *Taking Part in Community Care Planning.* Leeds/Edinburgh, Nuffield Institute for Health/Age Concern Scotland.

Rhodes, P., Nocon, A. (1998). User involvement and the NHS reforms. *Health Expectations,* 1: 73–81.

Saunders, C. (1998). Quoted in Commitments on caring for cancer. In *Information Exchange, National Council for Hospice and Specialist Palliative Care Services.* London, 25 June, pp. 6–7.

Small, N. (1989). *Politics and Planning in the National Health Service.* Milton Keynes, Open University Press.

Small, N. (2000). The modern hospice movement: 'bright lights sparkling' or 'a bit of heaven for a few'? In Bornat, J., Perks, R., Thompson, P., Walnsley, J. *Oral history, health and welfare.* London, Routledge, pp. 288–308.

Small, N., Rhodes, P. (2000). *Too Ill to Talk? User Involvement in Palliative Care.* London, Routledge.

Taylor, H. (1983). *The Hospice Movement in Britain: its role and its Functions.* London, Centre for Policy on Ageing.

Webster, C. (1998). *The National Health Service: A Political History.* Oxford, Oxford University Press.

3

Developments in user organizations

Jane Bradburn

Introduction

User involvement is a feature of health service policy in the UK. Discovering the needs and views of people who use health services and involving them in decision making about service developments and improvements has been actively promoted within the National Health Service (NHS). This policy imperative tends to obscure the impact that users themselves and in particular user organizations are making to get their voices heard. This chapter describes the growth of the user movement and the contribution this has made to giving a 'voice to the voiceless'. It then explores the way in which cancer user organizations in particular have developed user involvement alongside the NHS initiatives and describes some current developments, highlighting some of the issues relating to palliative care services user involvement and offering examples of good practice.

Who is the user?

We are all potential users of health services. The term 'user' of services could therefore include everyone. However here it is taken to include patients, carers, family, friends, advocates, members of organizations representing users' interests, 'hard to reach' and community groups and members of the public.

Users have been described as follows.

> People who have a unique expertise and perspective acquired from their experience of using health services or living with a disease or condition.
>
> (Fletcher and Bradburn 2000)

People who have a professional role in the health services (such as doctor, nurse or researcher) may also be users of cancer services. However people who do not also have a 'professional' role have a distinct and complementary role to play in the development of services. They can provide clarity of view about user issues unclouded by the many competing issues health professionals constantly have to juggle with.

User involvement in the context of palliative care

User involvement in the context of palliative care services includes all levels of care from the one-to-one relationship between patient or carer and health professional to service and policy developments. It can mean

◆ listening to users' experiences;

◆ empowering users to advocate on their own behalf;

◆ working with user groups in partnership.

On a one-to-one level it may mean health professionals, researchers and others listening to patients' views about using services and advocating on their behalf. However health professionals' representation should not be seen as a substitute for users representing themselves.

User involvement can mean empowering individuals and groups of users to have their own voice and advocate on their own behalf. Health professionals can become expert advisers which means that the patient or carer takes a passive role or they can develop an active partnership where users are involved in decision making, as the Table 3.1 demonstrates.

Table 3.1 Relationships between patients and health professionals

Expert adviser	Active partnership
Defines patient's needs	Elicits patient's needs
Gives advice	Discusses options
Solves problems for patient	Explores solutions with patient
Decides what information patient needs	Asks patient what information they want
Encourages dependency	Empowers and enables patient to develop confidence

Fletcher and Buggins (2000).

It is only by empowering the individual in meeting their own care needs that user involvement at all levels can be achieved. At a basic level this can be through giving people access to information. For example the National Cancer Alliance's TeamWork project has produced a patient folder with information relating to their cancer journey (National Cancer Alliance 2000). This folder, developed following focus group consultation with users, is a personal file of information about their care and treatment.

Levels of user involvement

The following model has been widely used to understand the different levels of user involvement (Hanley *et al.* 2000):

◆ consultation

◆ collaboration

◆ user control.

Methods for consulting users include contact by telephone, post and face to face; surveys, focus groups, panels and committees; and discussions with existing self-help and support or community groups. Consultation is a process in which the consulting authority sets the agenda. The choice of method will depend on the purpose of the exercise. Survey methods, for example, would be appropriate if it is important to know the views of a representative sample of service users, whilst consultations with existing groups might provide quick feedback on emerging issues. Focus groups have been used to collect patient and carer views to feed into the development of cancer services. They enable the user to set their own agenda but they do require skilled facilitators.

Users have been co-opted onto working groups and committees as patient and carer representatives, for example, as members of medical education and research committees including the Royal College of Physicians and the Consumer Liaison Group of the National Cancer Research Institute. Lone users on committees of health professionals have experienced significant difficulties in being actively involved and it is good practice for there to be at least two user representatives.

A number of cancer user groups (users and carers) or partnership groups (users, carers and health professionals) exist. These groups meet together to give the views of local patients and carers to local cancer services, commissioners and providers. They undertake a range of activities and are often members of other related committees. There are examples of such groups, facilitated either by a cancer network or hospital or community-based cancer resource centres (Miles and Jackson 1997).

Concerns are often expressed about how representative users are. Users cannot represent all other patients and carers just as doctors cannot represent the views of all other doctors. However, user representatives are encouraged to represent not simply their own individual views but also those of other people affected by cancer in the local community. For example, the Northamptonshire Partnership Forum are a group of user representatives trained in basic research methods who used questionnaires in order to access the views of current cancer service users. One obstacle for user representatives has been that this may require ethical approval and written patient consent, a process that they may be unfamiliar with and find daunting. Some user representatives rely on more informal methods of accessing user views, for example, talking to other members of their self-help group. Users with existing links to other patients and carers such as self-help and support group members can therefore make a valuable contribution.

Methods used to involve users vary according to the level of involvement, ranging from passive to more active methods. Partnership activities are those where users not only input their views but also actively participate with professionals in the plans resulting from that participation. A range of different methods can be matched to tasks and people can participate at different levels depending on their inclination and ability (Table 3.2).

User organizations

User or patient organizations have played and continue to play an important part in user involvement. Many of these organizations were started by concerned individuals themselves affected by a disease or illness for which they found little support. Motivated by this experience they set up small groups or organizations some of which grew and developed into national organizations (Wann 1995).

In the UK there are a large number of national voluntary organizations or non-governmental organizations representing the interests of specific patient groups with palliative care needs. Examples are the Multiple Sclerosis Society, Macmillan Cancer Relief and theTerrence Higgins Trust. There also exist a very large number of self-help groups some of which are branches of the larger national organizations and some of which are local independent and autonomous groups. The development of individual self-help groups depends on the needs and aspirations of members and this leads to a range of activities and forms of organization.

These organizations have in the past mainly focused on providing support to people affected by the condition. However the growth of the consumer

Table 3.2 User involvement: Levels, Methods, and Tasks

Level of involvement	Methods	Task
Informed	Newsletters, leaflets, posters, radio	Informing patients about entitlements, resources, new services or drugs
Consultation	Focus or discussion groups, semi-structured interviews, questionnaires	Finding out views on services
Collaboration/ partnership	Committees, working groups	Agreeing priorities for service improvements or research projects and carrying these out including feedback
User control	Self help and support groups, user groups	Users decide on priorities and action in response to their needs

and activist movements in the 1980s combined with the emphasis on self-help and self-advocacy has seen these groups become increasingly political. Groups have played a significant part in influencing policy largely as a result of social movements like the women's movement with respect to the growth in breast cancer advocacy and the gay movement with respect to HIV and Aids (Bradburn and Maher 1995).

Experiential knowledge

Government policy supporting user involvement and advocacy has focused attention on the potential of self-help groups to contribute their knowledge of a specific illness or condition to the improvement of health services and research. Borkman (1999) uses the term 'experiential truth' to distinguish the knowledge self-help group members gain through their personal experience of a disease or condition from 'professional truth' based on knowledge developed, applied and transmitted by an established specialized occupation by means of training or specialized education.

Experiential knowledge locates an expert knowledge with the patient or carer rather than locating expertise solely with the doctor or nurse.

Box 3.1 Listening to people's experiences

How people feel

'You have to take each day at a time because you can't look too far ahead because it would frighten you to death.'

What their attitudes are

'I have got to the stage now where I don't want to go to the MS Society because I am the worst.'

How they experience services and care

'A social worker's help was offered at the time ... I thought "Well, does he mean a counsellor or someone who is going to give me some encouragement?" But when it worked out, it seemed the social worker was coming to tell me all the benefits a disabled person could get.'

(Small and Rhodes 2000)

People with experiential knowledge can contribute to understanding the experience of a condition by telling us how they feel, their attitudes and how they respond to the care services they receive (Box 3.1).

Linking support and influence

Research has demonstrated how experiential knowledge generated by groups can be used by its members to influence health service policy thus linking support to advocacy. For example, individuals from a network of local cancer support groups decided that they wanted to have a voice in local decisions about service delivery of cancer care (Bradburn and Mackie 2001). The group used their knowledge to contribute to local decision making by becoming user representatives on local health committees implementing changes to cancer services following proposals in the Calman Hine Report (Department of Health 1995). Similarly Barnes describes how a group of mental health users used their experiential knowledge to contribute to service development in mental health services (Barnes and Shardlow 1997).

The term 'user group' is now used to refer to people who have experience of using health services either as a patient or carer and who have come together to use that knowledge in order to influence the services.

There is some confusion about the terms applied to groups of people who use cancer services, 'patient groups', 'self-help groups', 'consumer groups', 'voluntary groups' and so on. Self-help and support groups have the primary purpose of offering emotional and practical support to people affected by the provision of services. The term 'user group' refers to people who have experience of using cancer services either as patients or carers and who have come together to use that knowledge in order to influence the provision of cancer services.

User groups are developing across the UK, largely as a result of government policy, which encourages user involvement. Many of these groups are working with hospitals and primary care groups to improve local services. User representatives work at local, regional and national levels. They can be specific to a disease or condition, for example, breast cancer or include users with experiences of different diseases or conditions. User groups may include members of self-help and support groups but they may also include individuals and include other advocates. They often work as members of joint committees and forums with health professionals and managers.

What part do user groups play in supportive and palliative care?

User involvement is an important part of ensuring quality in supportive care services. There are many examples of user groups working effectively in this way. For example, the Rotherham Cancer Users Forum undertook a survey of patient information in general practitioners' surgeries, which highlighted the need for more information about cancer being displayed in the surgeries.

Users may act as advocates on behalf of others who do not have the confidence to ask questions or put forward their views, for example, by accompanying a patient to a consultation with their doctor. An example of this kind of activity is that provided for cancer service users and their families by the Liverpool Cancer Support Centre (Box 3.2).

Users may also offer their services as volunteers in the supportive care services offered by the NHS. They may be members of self-help groups who set up and run services themselves. This often happens where users identify gaps in services or find that the current NHS services do not meet their needs or those of other users and carers. For example, Bosom Friends, a breast cancer group in Hillingdon, were instrumental in setting up a community drop-in centre where people could easily access cancer information and support.

Box 3.2 Liverpool Cancer Support Centre

This is a user run, managed and led service providing practical, emotional and psychological support to people affected by cancer in Merseyside. The Centre's services are firmly based around an ethos of advocacy, mainly self-advocacy, but also peer group support and limited professional support. A 'focus group', which is regularly attended by 15 to 20 people each week with people at different stages of diagnosis, treatment and care, discusses issues. The more established members provide support to newer members with minimal input from facilitators. The Centre encourages people to advocate on their own behalf to health professionals providing their care. It believes that everyone has different skills and strengths and that they just need some support to refine those skills following diagnosis and then to use them in new ways in the future.

(Keatley and Berry 2002)

Building capacity

In the UK there are many user organizations that support people with an experience of cancer. Unlike many other countries the UK does not have a single Cancer Society. Organizations have emerged in response to need; some focus on specific cancers, for example, breast, ovarian and kidney and others have a broader focus. For example, Cancerlink (now part of Macmillan Cancer Relief) offers support to the over 600 cancer self-help and support groups in the UK. Groups continue to be set up and to disappear, the sector is constantly changing in response to people's needs. The diverse nature of the sector means that there is a choice of organizations offering different kinds of support. However this has also hindered building a strong user voice in cancer services. See Box 3.3.

The capacity-building requirements of users and carers has been recognized through a number of research studies. The need for training for user representatives working in a range of different settings has been shown to be important (Bradburn *et al.* 2000). User representatives often find that they lack confidence when they are part of a committee comprising health professionals. Some may be unfamiliar with committees and with the organization of the health services. Consumers in NHS Research, a standing advisory group that promotes user or consumer involvement, has produced

Box 3.3 Cancer VOICES Project, Macmillan Cancer Relief

'CancerVOICES' is an independent network of cancer services user representatives supported by Macmillan Cancer Relief. CancerVOICES provides support and training to user representatives so that they can work effectively with health professionals. Training developed for lay members of Maternity Service Liaison Committees was piloted through the VOICES in ACTION Project and has been used successfully to train cancer service users as part of the CancerVOICES Project. The training is linked to support, information and networking.

(Bradburn 2001*a*)

guidelines for researchers and for users. Training courses for users have been developed by CancerVOICES at Macmillan Cancer Relief, the College of Health and the Public Health Research Unit, Oxford.

User involvement in cancer services

User involvement in the NHS is high on the cancer services policy agenda. The Calman Hine Report set out a plan for the re-organization of cancer services and recommended that cancer services should be 'patient-centred'. Following publication of the report, cancer services in England are now organized into 34 cancer networks. These are networks of hospitals, hospices and primary care trusts, together with all those organizations caring for cancer patients, working together with the aim of providing seamless, quality services. Each cancer network is managed by a lead manager, lead clinician and lead nurse with an executive board and steering group.

User involvement is a priority for these networks.

> At a local level, cancer networks will be expected to take account of the views of patients and carers when planning services.
>
> (Department of Health 2001).

This development is mirrored by the development of palliative and supportive care networks that are being established to link together organizations and care staff providing care.

The National Cancer Task Force has developed guidance on how users can be involved in cancer services (Bradburn 2001*b*). This recognizes that to be really effective, user involvement needs to be integral to the development and organization of cancer services at all levels (national, regional and local) rather than to run parallel to it with the danger it might become marginalized and tokenistic.

The approach suggested is of cancer partnership groups set up in each cancer network. The concept is similar to the existing maternity service liaison committees in maternity services, which exist in hospital trusts.

The groups are an integral part of the structure of each cancer network and comprise equal numbers of health professionals and users. Their role is to facilitate and advise on user involvement for the whole cancer network and to raise local patient issues for the network to address. They provide a pool of cancer service user representatives from different backgrounds and with experience of different cancers, who can work with a variety of committees and working groups within the network. At least two users should be members of the executive board and steering group for the network. Partnership groups and user groups are already linking with multi-disciplinary teams and tumour-specific groups as well as the patient liaison advisory services set up under the government's patient and public involvement initiative. They also link to the wider community through existing links with voluntary sector organizations and patient or user groups.

Traditionally user involvement in cancer services has been located within supportive and palliative care. The approach recognizes that user involvement cannot and should not be pigeon-holed but should apply to all parts of the cancer services including clinical areas and supportive and palliative care networks.

Lack of research evidence on user involvement in cancer services is currently being addressed by a three-year Department of Health-funded research programme by the Avon, Somerset and Wiltshire Cancer Project, which will shortly be completed. Early evidence from the project indicates the value of a joint user/professional forum to advise and facilitate user involvement within the cancer network.

A voice for palliative care services

In spite of these developments there are still barriers to the involvement of palliative care service users. There is the concern that palliative care services users may be too ill and should not be asked to spend time answering questionnaires as this might detract from their quality of life in the time left to them. However recent research challenging this view has shown that although palliative care users might be few in number, their needs were great and those needs were different from the wider population and required services from a range of agencies (Small and Rhodes 2000). Talking to their carers was not a substitute as their needs might be quite different from the carer but equally as important. The research showed that people with terminal illnesses did sometimes want to contribute to changes in services that would be put in place after they were no longer alive, seeing this as their legacy to others. However the researchers cautioned that palliative care service users might have other priorities than taking part in research.

Other barriers to palliative care service user involvement are the practical obstacles to collective forms of participation. These include the uncertainty about how they will feel on the day, the need for reliable transport, a suitable venue and a format that is not too tiring (Beresford *et al.* 2000*a*).

For people from different ethnic groups the barriers may be more complex. Research shows that the number of black and ethnic minority people using hospice and palliative care services is low in proportion to their numbers (Hill and Penso 1995). Communication and cultural sensitivity are important factors but the role of advocates, interpreters and link workers who can speak up for and support individuals is very important. Health advocates can lead to users having greater confidence about using services (Mount 2001).

Involving palliative care users requires an understanding of the practical, emotional and psychological issues they face. The familiar ways of involving users such as committees may not be the best given these considerations. What is required is imaginative ways of involving users. There are a growing number of good practice examples in palliative care service user involvement.

First national seminar on patient/user involvement in palliative care

The first national seminar on patient/user involvement in palliative care was held at St Christopher's Hospice, Education Centre, London and funded by the Joseph Rowntree Foundation. The majority of participants were service users so that they could feel they had the key role in the day and that their views were really valued. Presentations were kept short so that the day was not tiring and there was plenty of opportunity for discussion. Key issues that emerged included the importance of maximizing people's control over their lives, of self-help and support groups and of meaningful involvement rather than tokenism. Participants wanted more opportunities for meeting together and a national group has now been set up (Beresford *et al.* 2000*b*).

St Christopher's Hospice

At St Christopher's Hospice, two user groups have been successfully set up, one for ward-based patients and one for those living at home. Both are held at the hospice. Great attention is paid to the practical aspects of the meetings; transport is provided, group discussion sessions are short, a nurse is available and toilets accessible. Meetings are held three times a year. Not all people attending one meeting may be able to make the next, some may be too ill and some may have died. Effective and prompt feedback and action on issues raised is therefore prioritized. A senior member of the hospice staff as well as the coordinator attends meetings. Issues raised by the groups are taken to clinical management meetings and staff responsible for the area involved undertake to put changes into action where this is possible and appropriate. This is then fed back to the users by letter as well as verbally in meetings.

The Beacon Project

The Beacon Project in Brighton, which provides care for people with HIV and Aids, has a user forum, set up to enable users to express their views about service provision and to put forward ideas and discuss issues. Members are drawn mainly from day care users and meet bi-monthly. As an advisory body within the Beacon, the forum has the power to make recommendations to the management and has a representative on the Council of Management as a full trustee. Members hold their own meeting first to discuss their issues and then invite the staff into the meeting. Then whichever member of staff is responsible for the issue raised deals with it. The issues raised by the forum concern the services provided by the centre and include such topics as access to transport, food and funding. The forum has led to closer collaboration between service users and staff and services better tailored to meet ongoing needs. The forum won the National Council of Hospices Award for user involvement initiatives in 2001 (National Council for Hospice and Specialist Palliative Care Services 2001a).

The Candle Project

The Candle Project at St Christopher's Hospice includes a self-help group set up by two users who as bereaved parents felt there was a need for support to others like themselves. It meets about five times a year to talk about their issues. The group provides parents with a quiet time away from their children where feelings can be discussed openly. Transport is available together with quality on-site childcare provided by Candle Project volunteers. Members are able to share their grief safely. Topics discussed include practical issues, caring for grieving children and making new relationships. Referrals come through staff of the Candle Project at St Christopher's Hospice and the group has maintained a diverse ethnic, class and gender mix. Feedback from the group has proved the value of a group of peers with which to share experiences and difficult issues (National Council for Hospice and Specialist Palliative Care Services 2001b).

The Dorothy House Hospice Care Service

The Dorothy House Hospice Care Service has involved their service users in a range of different ways. They have involved users through their clinical audit programme. Patient satisfaction surveys using questionnaires to patients attending day care and the in-patient unit are regularly carried out. A questionnaire for the bereaved has been used to find out views about the bereavement service and a user is involved as part of the bereavement working party.

An audit of patients using complementary therapies found that while 50% of patients had died over the period audited, 24 out of 38 questionnaires sent to suitable patients were returned. The audit identified the need for patients and staff to have more information about the therapies offered. A leaflet for patients has now been written and awareness-raising sessions for staff are planned.

A focus group meeting was held to review day care with 10 current patients, one discharged patient and one carer. They were divided into smaller groups and asked to say what was helpful about coming to day care and what was the most difficult thing. As a larger group they looked at the kind of changes they would like to see. The main themes for change were more support and information for carers, more information and a patient's newsletter. A focus group meeting was also held to assist with web site development, which gave guidance about important features for its design and content (National Council for Hospice and Specialist Palliative Care Services 2002).

Other quite different and less intrusive approaches may be more appropriate for people whose degree of illness precludes collective user involvement approaches. For example, the Gold Standards Framework Project for Community and Palliative Care, a joint Macmillan Cancer Relief and NHS Modernisation Agency initiative, provides a home pack for patients or carers to keep at home. The pack includes useful information on caring and living with cancer at home, key contacts and a weekly review sheet. This sheet can be used by the patient or carer to feed back problems or gaps in care to those caring for them so that these can be addressed immediately where possible. The views given by patient and carer can also be used to improve services for others. The pack is written in accessible language and clearly set out and enables the individual user to be involved in improving care both for themselves and others (Thomas 2001).

This kind of approach confers direct benefit to the individual while also collecting information about user need more generally.

Conclusion

User organizations play an important role in enabling people to have a voice. Sharing their experience and issues as a peer group can confer confidence and a shared identity and build knowledge. Users' experience and knowledge of services are important in order to develop more integrated and patient-centred services. Confident users can also challenge our perceptions. It is dangerous to assume that just because people have crossed a line between active and palliative care, they are not well enough to take an active part in user involvement. This kind of stereotyping only serves to mirror the divide users themselves often experience when moving from active treatment to palliative care which can mean a change in the staff they see or the places that they go for treatment. Palliative care service users are actively involved in a wide range of activities including membership of cancer network partnership groups, user groups and self-help groups.

User involvement in palliative care services does present particular challenges but there are now a number of examples of good practice that indicate that service users can and are willing to have their voices heard. These include questionnaires to obtain feedback about services, focus groups to find out user views as well as self-help and user groups. Many of these examples are located within local hospice services. The challenge for the future, as more people are expected to be supported at home, is to develop approaches that extend to primary care and community services.

There are real barriers to involving those who are very ill and yet they are often the ones who rely most heavily on services. We need imaginative approaches to overcome these barriers, which rely less on the collective and traditional research methods and which result in speedy action where this is needed to benefit both the individual and the wider population of users.

Finally the example of how user involvement has been built into cancer services shows that to be really effective, user involvement needs to be integral to the development and organization of services. It needs to be adequately resourced at all levels if it is to avoid being tokenistic so that users have an effective voice which truly influences services.

References

Barnes M and Shardlow P (1997) From passive recipient to active citizen: participation in mental health groups. Journal of Mental Health 6, 289–300.

Beresford P, Croft S and Oliviere D (2002a) Our Lives, not our Illness. Briefing Number 6, November 2000. London: National Council for Hospice and Specialist Palliative Care Services.

Beresford P, Broughton F, Craft S, Oliviere D, and Rhodes, P (2000b) Palliative Care: Developing User Involvement, Improving Quality. Report of the First National Seminar of Palliative Care Service Users and Workers, St Christopher's Education Centre, Sydenham. The Centre for Citizen Participation, Middlesex: Brunel University.

Borkman T (1999) Understanding Self-help and Mutual Aid: Experiential Learning in the Commons. New Jersey: Rutgers University Press.

Bradburn J (2001a) Listening to the voices of experience. Professional Nurse 16 (Supplement).

Bradburn J (2001b) User involvement in cancer services. Report to the National Cancer Task Force (unpublished).

Bradburn J and Mackie C (2001) Action research with cancer service users. In A Handbook for Action Research in Health and Social Care, Winter R and Munn-Giddings C (ed.). London: Routledge.

Bradburn J and Maher J (1995) The growth of advocacy groups for cancer patients in Europe and the USA. Oncology Today 12, 14–17.

Bradburn J, Fletcher G and Kennelly C (2000) Voices in Action Research Report. London: College of Health.

Department of Health (1995) A Policy Framework for Commissioning Cancer Services (The Calman Hine Report). London: Department of Health/HMSO.

Department of Health (2001) The National Cancer Plan. London: Department of Health/HMSO.

Fletcher G and Bradburn J (2000) Voices in Action Resource Book. London: College of Health.

Fletcher G and Buggins E (2000) Midwifery Practice Care Topic 3: Empowerment a Gift Bestowed or Withheld? London: Macmillan Press.

Hanley B, Bradburn J, Gorin S, Barnes M, Evans C, Goodane H, Kelson M, Kent A, Oliver S, and Wallcraft, J (2000) Involving Consumers in Research and

Development in the NHS: Briefing Notes for Researchers. Winchester: Consumers in NHS Research Support Unit.

Hill D and Penso D (1995) Opening Doors: Improving Access to Hospice and Specialist Palliative Care Services by Members of the Black and Ethnic Minority Communities. Occasional Paper 7. London: National Council for Hospice and Specialist Palliative Care Services.

Keatley S and Berry S (2002) Advocacy project. Unpublished report of the Liverpool Cancer Support Centre.

Miles R and Jackson R (1997) Involving Local Cancer Service Users in Planning and Developing Cancer Services: a Feasibility Study. Report to East Sussex, Brighton and Hove Health Authority. Oxford: National Cancer Alliance.

Mount J (2001) Palliative Care Services for Different Ethnic Groups: Proceedings of a Seminar held in December 2000. London: National Council for Hospice and Specialist Palliative Care Services.

National Cancer Alliance (2000) TeamWork Project. Oxford: National Cancer Alliance.

National Council for Hospice and Specialist Palliative Care Services (2001a) Views of clients are crucial in running of care centre. Information Exchange Number 33, September p. 10.

National Council for Hospice and Specialist Palliative Care Services (2001b) Parents' group shares experience. Information Exchange Number 33, September, p. 10.

National Council for Hospice and Specialist Palliative Care Services (2002) Patients and carers take part in developing services. Information Exchange, Number 35, May, pp. 12–13.

Small N and Rhodes P (2000) Too Ill To Talk: User Involvement in Palliative Care. London: Routledge.

Thomas K (2001) The Gold Standards Framework Project for Community Palliative Care Home Pack: Information for Patients and Carers. London: Macmillan Cancer Relief and the NHS Modernisation Agency.

Wann M (1995) Building Social Capital: Self Help in the Twenty-First Century Welfare State. London: Institute of Public Policy Research.

4

Quality issues in palliative and supportive care

Sam H. Ahmedzai and John Hunt

Introduction

In addressing the issues of 'quality' in the care of people with a limited life-span, it is important first of all to distinguish the two main areas that are relevant for palliative care. These are first, 'quality of life' of patients and their carers and second, 'quality of care' delivered by services. Often in casual discussion these two aspects are confused and blurred, with a resulting loss of precision of meaning, and consequently of their practical implications. Indeed, it has been pointed out that 'one of the major problems, however, [in determining what constitutes quality care for the dying] in making such a determination results from the lack of consensus regarding a conceptual definition of quality' (Thompson and McClement 2002).

Quality of life in healthcare is often construed as a predominantly clinical concept, and in the past it has indeed been defined and measured in terms that reflect more the doctors' priorities than those of the users of services. Thus in the field of oncology, clinical trials in the late 1980s and early 1990s started to use quality of life as a (mainly secondary) end-point of trials employing new anti-cancer therapies. Initially this was measured using performance status instruments such as the Karnofsky scale (Karnofsky and Burchenal 1949). This scale in fact measures mobility and independent activity, on a range from fully mobile and capable of working, to totally bedbound and fully dependent on nursing help. Although this could be a useful measure of the physical capability of patients and the degree of nursing and social services they require, it tells us very little of the personal experience of the individuals and their perceived quality of life. It is of course entirely possible for a person to be totally paralysed and dependent on help, but still maintain a sense of psychological coherence and self-worth, and to be a loved and valued member of a family and community (Twycross 1987). There have been many well-conducted empirical studies that have explored the differences in the users' and their professionals' (mainly doctors and nurses) viewpoints on the nature and breadth of quality of life. Generally speaking, these studies have shown that professionals tend to under-estimate physical symptoms and psychosocial distress; but they can also under-estimate the value that patients place on their own overall quality of life. Similarly, although family carers can have greater insight into a patient's distress, studies have also shown that their ratings too do not always accord with the patient's (O'Brien and Francis 1988; Ahmedzai *et al.* 1988).

During the late 1980s there was, however, a move towards developing quality-of-life concepts that tapped more broadly into the multidimensional nature of the individual's perception of what gave their life quality. Thus the European Organisation for Research and Treatment of Cancer (EORTC)— a major European collaborative cancer research group—initiated a line of studies with the aim of capturing—using self-reported questionnaires—the cancer patient's own perspective on quality of life before and after treatment (Aaronson *et al.* 1988). In the USA, the Rand Corporation initiated research on a more generic way of measuring quality of life, which could apply to a variety of diagnostic groups and which has led to the SF-36 instrument (Ware *et al.* 1994). The most recent methodology to be developed has taken the user perspective even further, and is based on a more open-ended interaction between user and researcher, using an interview that explores the person's own determinants of quality of life (McGee *et al.* 1991). These approaches will be discussed and appraised in more detail below.

The second aspect of 'quality' highlighted at the start of this section was quality of care as provided by services. The process of focusing on and improving on quality of care is known as quality assurance. Of course, quality of life and quality of care are logically closely related concepts: quality of care offered by a service should impact directly on the quality of life experienced by the user, and the measured quality of life of users should influence changes in services. However, in practice it is helpful to consider them separately. There are two main reasons for this: first, because quality of care is concerned primarily with the *structure and process* of healthcare interventions whilst quality of life represents primarily the *outcome*, using the language of healthcare evaluation introduced by Donabedian (1980). Seen this way, both concepts therefore represent a continuum of opportunities to measure and give feedback on the user–provider interaction.

The second reason for separating the two issues is that professionals now acknowledge, with greater humility than before, that there are many more aspects of a person's and family's quality of life than can be influenced by, or even known to, a health or social care service. This can be demonstrated in drug studies of new palliative interventions. A UK multicentre random-ized controlled trial of cancer pain control clearly demonstrated that a new therapy (a novel way of delivering an analgesic drug using a three-day skin patch, compared to conventional twice daily tablets) was associated with numerous advantages which could be measured in terms of symptoms, side-effects, convenience and overall preference (Ahmedzai and Brooks 1997). Thus, the *quality of care* to these patients was undoubtedly improved by the new therapy; their views in these respects were mirrored by their clinicians' estimates of improved symptom control. However, when the same patients who reported these benefits were asked to comment on their *quality of life*, using a reputable standardized questionnaire, there was no difference between the periods of time they were receiving the two medica-tions. This suggests that the make-up of these patients' quality of life was more complex than the sum of symptom control and convenience of med-ication; or put another way, while medical care can have a significant impact on the externally measurable aspects of daily life, the concurrent changes in a person's quality of life remains private—and perhaps, ulti-mately inscrutable.

Which aspect of quality is 'right'?

Which is the more important concept in palliative care? We would argue that both are equally valid and indeed are so inter-related that both should be incorporated into a comprehensive evaluation of the quality of any form of health and social care. For palliative and supportive care for people with life-limiting diseases, this two-pronged approach is essential. It is widely accepted that one of the chief goals of palliative care is improving, or at least maintaining, the quality of life for patients and their carers (WHO 1990). Since those who are the prime recipients of palliative care tend to be physically less able to communicate their views, especially towards the ter-minal stage of illness, it is incumbent on palliative care services to make the extra effort of using different ways of capturing their perceptions.

Figure 4.1 shows diagrammatically how quality of care and quality of life can be seen to encompass the entire spectrum of assessment of palliative care delivery. In this chapter we will illustrate this model by describing and critiquing instruments that cover this whole range. Taking cancer care as an

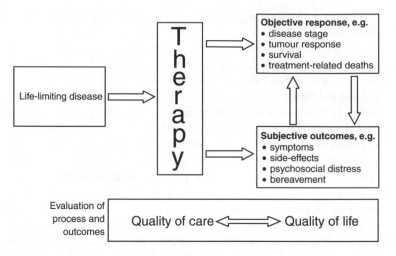

Fig. 4.1 Relationship of quality of care and quality of life to the therapeutic process and outcomes.

example, the treatments for the disease include surgery, chemotherapy, radiotherapy and hormone therapy. Common assessments of the quality of care associated with these therapies include waiting times, communication between patients and staff, and user satisfaction with clinics. In an institution such as a hospice or in a hospital palliative care department, structure and process measures such as the number of staff available, their level of training and how well they interact with users, are also measurable quality-of-care markers. Yet more examples are details such as the catering, parking facilities and availability of private rooms for carers to visit patients and for meetings with staff. A comprehensive quality-of-care assessment therefore needs to take all of these into consideration, although it will usually focus on specific areas during a particular evaluation exercise.

The outcomes of cancer care are divided in Fig. 4.1 into two groups: objective and subjective. Chronic disease management should ideally be directed at both of these, as both are important for the patients' lives. Typically, clinicians are more inclined to measure the objective outcomes such as changing disease stage, measurable changes in the disease (for example, tumour size in cancer, left ventricular ejection fraction in heart failure), length of overall survival and the numbers of patients who die as a result of treatment. Palliative care has not usually been involved with measuring these aspects of the patients' disease. However, oncology, cardiology and palliative care services should all be interested in the second set of outcomes, which are concerned with the patients' and carers' subjective experiences. These include physical symptoms, side-effects of both the disease-directed and purely palliative treatments, levels of psychosocial functioning and distress and the occurrence of abnormal bereavement. Recently, palliative care researchers have also tried to measure spiritual concerns and changes in these during the patients' illness.

Figure 4.1 shows that the objective and subjective changes can interact with each other. Lack of response to anti-cancer therapy is thus usually associated with worsening symptoms and often psychosocial distress. Side-effects of surgery or chemotherapy can have a major impact on patients' length of life but also their physical and social functioning. In the opposite direction, intolerable side-effects can lead some patients to withdraw early from anti-cancer treatment, which could adversely affect their survival time. Similarly, untreated psychological distress during treatment, not necessarily related to the actual therapy but possibly due to unrecognized domestic stress, could influence how long other patients persist with anti-cancer treatment. Thus, the combination of objective and subjective outcomes is linked into a comprehensive or holistic concept of quality of life, which is itself inextricably tied in with the length of remaining life.

Some quality-of-life researchers have tried to express these links in mathematical constructs, which gives a better impression of how good the quality of extra life gained with life-prolonging therapy has been for the patients. One simple measure is 'symptom-free survival', which is the length of life before symptoms recur after primary treatment; another more sophisticated approach is Q-TWiST, which stands for 'quality of time without symptoms of disease or toxicity of treatment' (Gelber *et al.* 1998). This complex, statistically derived outcome measure has been used to give greater insight into the benefits compared to the drawbacks of anti-cancer or HIV treatment. So far these techniques have not been explored as fully in non-cancer terminal diseases apart from AIDS, and they have not been applied to purely palliative treatments. It could be argued that as palliative care is not concerned with prolonging life, then such measures are not necessary. On the other hand it could be countered that, even if extra length of life is not the intention, it would be harmful to patients if palliative treatments reduced the quality of remaining time, and we would therefore argue that palliative care should, in the future, apply itself more rigorously to these kind of integrative objective–subjective measures.

In Fig. 4.1 an arrow is seen going between quality-of-care and quality-of-life measurement, in both directions. This connection between the two

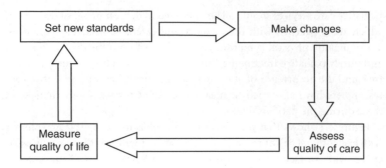

Fig. 4.2 The quality improvement cycle—how users' view of care and quality of life can influence delivery of care.

concepts reflects the principles of the quality improvement cycle, which is expanded in Fig. 4.2. In this model, quality-of-life assessment generates new information about the experience of end-users relating to a particular therapy or kind of service, for example, a recently instituted home care team. Feeding this information back to the staff involved in managing and delivering the treatment or service should help them initiate changes in how these are given in the future, and to set new higher standards for future organization of care. Quality-of-care assessment also helps by giving feedback to senior management on how the structure and process of care is perceived by users and clinical staff.

User involvement in measuring quality

How can users influence the processes described in Figs 4.1 and 4.2? It has already been argued that quality-of-life outcomes can only be measured by direct consultation with users. That is clearly the ideal situation, but what happens when patients become too ill and weak, confused or just tired of answering questions, as inevitably most will in palliative care? One response to this situation is to turn instead to the carers, and ask them the questions. Previous studies have shown that whilst carers can indeed act as proxies for the patients they know, their responses can systematically under-estimate or over-estimate some problems as compared to patients' own estimates. This issue was revisited in a recent study that was concerned with the validation of Quality of End-of-life Care and Satisfaction with Treatment (QUEST), a new instrument for measuring satisfaction with end-of-life care (Sulmasy *et al.* 2002). Here the researchers found a moderate correlation between patients' and their carers' ratings on quality of medical care, but there were no significant correlations for quality of nursing care, nor for satisfaction with either medical or nursing care.

Another possibility is to ask the staff's view of the patients' symptoms and other quality-of-life outcomes. Again, it has been shown that nurses as well as doctors can misjudge the scope and severity of problems compared to the patients' view (Heaven and McGuire 1997). These differences, which are found in research settings, might not be so evident in routine palliative care, where staff who have been involved with the patients remain in continuity, and where relationships build up between staff and carers, who gradually take over speaking on behalf of the patients as they become progressively ill.

However the differences between patient and staff or carer as proxies can have a significant impact in research, where greater bias-free precision is required. It is also of higher relevance in the case of patients who are unable to communicate with professionals from the outset of their illness, for example, because of mental problems such as dementia, speech difficulties such as dysphasia after stroke or inability of the patients or carers to speak the language of the professional team. In the former cases, it may be necessary to rely on the views of family carers, with the proviso that they should be close to the patient and preferably be living with them, or be familiar with their living conditions, for example, a spouse, or adult daughter or son of an older patient. In the last case, it is incumbent on the palliative care service to find a suitable interpreter who can mediate in the patient's own language. If a questionnaire is being used to measure quality of life, it is notable that very few of the quality measures described later in this chapter have been translated into many languages—the EORTC QLQ-C30 quality-of-life questionnaire is one notable example, as it is available in 23 languages at present.

Assuming that there is good communication between patients, carers and staff, how can service users influence the measurement of quality in palliative care? The first way is to work with the professionals in designing better quality measures. In Table 4.1, we have shown where the leading quality measures have benefited from user involvement in their design. Regrettably, this has not usually been the case, until recently. The second way is by participating in the collection of user views of both quality of care and quality of life. Whereas in the past it was considered acceptable for staff to make judgements about patients' and carers' experiences, for example, with the Support Team Assessment Schedule (STAS), the current instruments are

Table 4.1 Quality measures for palliative care: derivation, characteristics, and application of current instruments

Measure	Type*	Domains and items	Published criteria	Settings in which developed**	User involvement in development?	Applications	User completes (yes or no) (Proxy-Professional or carer)***	Registration/cost
Support Team Assessment Schedule (STAS)	Clinical	17 items. 10 patient and family, 7 service. 9 items for SPCUs.	Yes	Community palliative care teams (UK)	Yes—patients and carers	SPCUs and community	No Proxy—professional	Yes/none
Edmonton Symptom Assessment Schedule (ESAS)	Clinical	Symptom status. 10-item VAS relating to specific symptoms	Yes	SPCU (Canada)	No	SPCUs	Yes Proxy by nurses	No/free
Palliative Care Assessment (PACA)	Clinical	10 items covering 8 core symptoms, patient and carer insight and patient's future placement	Yes	Acute hospital (UK)	No	Acute hospital services	Yes	No/free
Palliative Care Outcome Scale (POS)	Clinical	12 items. Symptoms, patient/family anxiety, information, support, existential, performance status	Yes	SPCUs (UK)	No	SPCUs and community	Yes Professional	Yes/free

Views of Informal Carers—Evaluation of Services (VOICES)	Retrospective Clinical/Organizational	42 questions about care received in the last year of life, from a range of care providers (primary, secondary, specialist and social services)	Yes	Hospital, community and SPCUs (UK)	Yes—in piloting the original measure. Views of users/bereaved relatives used in the content and design of the new revised version (2002)	Postal questionnaire	Yes	Bereaved carer or person who knew the patient best during the last year of life	Yes	No fee currently. Likely to introduce a small cost to cover materials.****
Trent Hospice Audit Group (THAG)	Clinical/organizational	Clinical, educational and management. 7 standards: 4 audit packages containing 51 items	Yes	SPCUs (UK)	Yes—patients, carers and bereaved carers	SPCUs, acute and cancer hospitals, (nursing) care homes	Yes	Proxy—carer (specially designed form)	Yes/free, no fee currently. Likely to introduce charges in future	
Health Quality Service (HQS)	Organizational	Specific standards module for hospice services covering 4 sections: philosophy of care; hospice governance and management; the patient's experience and the environment for care	Yes	SPCUs (UK)		SPCUs cancer and acute hospitals, community			Yes/fees range from £4000 to £8000 for a 3-year accreditation cycle	

Table 4.1 Quality measures for palliative care: derivation, characteristics, and application of current instruments (*contd*)

Measure	Type*	Domains and items	Published criteria	Settings in which developed**	User involvement in development?	Applications	User completes (yes or no) (Proxy-Professional or carer)***	Registration/cost
Quality by Peer Review (QPR)	Organizational	3 core modules (Clinical, organizational and strategic). 7 consistent categories in each module, Total number of items unpublished	No	SPCUs in Yorkshire, UK	Yes	Hospice organizations. Use in community and specialist hospital palliative care teams being explored	Yes Both patients and carers, details unpublished	£3000 annual subscription fee and £2000 joining fee or £6500 and expenses for an individual audit
McGill Quality of Life Questionnaire (MQOL)	Quality of life/clinical	16 items. 4 subscales: physical symptoms; psychological symptoms; outlook on life; and meaningful existence	Yes	Cancer and acute hospital, SPCUs (Canada)	Yes	Cancer and acute hospital, SPCUs, community, AIDS clinic, pain clinic, ALS clinic	Yes	Yes/no cost if not being used for profit
European Organization for Research and Treatment of Cancer (EORTC) QLQ-C30	Quality of life/clinical	30 items: 9 multi-item scales; 5 functional scales; 3 symptom scales; several single item scales; and a global health and quality of life scale	Yes	Cancer hospital (international)	Yes—patient	Cancer hospitals	Yes Proxy—professional	Yes/free for academic/clinical use. Charges for commercially sponsored studies

Instrument	Domain	Description	*	Setting	***	Populations	Proxy	Cost
Quality of End-of-life Care and Satisfaction with Treatment (QUEST)	Quality of life/clinical	15 items covering perception of staff availability; attentiveness; bedside manner; courtesy; way of talking; clinical skills; and overall satisfaction	Yes	Teaching hospital—internal medicine (USA)	Yes—patients and 'surrogates'	Hospital	Yes Proxy—carer (surrogate)	No
Schedule for the Evaluation of Individual Quality of Life (SEIQoL)	Quality of life	Patients asked to nominate the 5 areas of life that they consider are most important to their QOL using a segmented coloured disc, to rate each domain using a vertical analogue scale and rate their global QOL	Yes	Acute hospital (UK and Ireland)	Yes—patient	SPCU, cancer and acute hospitals, community, healthy young, healthy elderly, carers, wide range of clinical populations	Yes	No/nominal cost to cover printing costs of the manual

* See text for codes.

** Specialist Palliative Care Units (SPCUs) include hospices.

*** Yes = patient fills in answers.

**** If the survey is used by a palliative care service there are no additional costs. However, there are charges otherwise, incurred by the need to use the Office of National Statistics services (currently £8 per death certificate).

asking similar questions but directly of the users, for example, the Palliative Outcome Scale (POS).

Some quality-of-care measures in hospital and hospice practice can be taken from case notes and medical records without direct patient involvement, for example, waiting times, but whenever a subjective view is required then the users' view should be sought. In Fig. 4.2, it can be seen that users can thus directly influence the two stages of measuring quality of care and measuring quality of life. Can users' roles be extended? We would argue that consumer consultation practices should in the future allow for users of services to become involved also in at least one other stage of Fig. 4.2. This is in the setting of new standards and procedures, whether they apply to waiting times, provision of ward or hospice facilities or to clinical interventions. An example of the latter could be consultation with users and their representatives when new protocols are being written, for example, for patient self-dispensing of medication in an in-patient unit or for a policy about the use of artificial hydration in terminally ill people. How could such views be obtained? One route is to collect data on the satisfaction with care and quality-of-life outcomes with new interventions. Morita and Adachi (2002) have shown this is possible even with very ill patients, who were receiving artificial hydration. Another approach could be to hold focus groups, or conduct surveys with current users and their representatives or with carers who have witnessed the intervention in question with the patient in the past and can comment on their view of its effects.

Recent policy developments in the measurement of quality

Before discussing the development of quality-of-care tools in palliative care *per se*, it is worth reflecting on their place in the overall context of quality assurance in the health and social care system. Chapter 2 has already covered in detail the policy issues surrounding the area of providing a voice for the consumers of healthcare. We wish to highlight in brief the important ways in which the UK Government has brought these issues to the attention of the public and professions, by a series of papers, starting with the Calman–Hine report (Calman and Hine 1995) on the need to re-organize cancer services. This very influential document paved the way for the centralization of cancer services in the UK, using the approach which has become known as the 'national service framework'. Part of the vision of Calman and Hine was to incorporate palliative care services into mainstream cancer care, rather than letting it be seen it as an 'optional extra' on the periphery.

The resulting NHS Cancer Plan (Department of Health 2000) has started to clarify how this is to be done, with specific recommendations on the structure and process of palliative care teams operating within cancer centres and cancer units, and also of those existing independently in hospices. The Cancer Plan did not, however, make specific recommendations about how the outcome of those services (that is, the quality of life that results for the users) could be measured. It remains to be seen if this will be addressed by other UK Government papers on both cancer and other disease areas, via the emerging stream of national service frameworks in the care of elderly people and people with heart disease, neurological disease, renal disease and so on.

A positive feature of recent UK Government policy in this area is the addition of a relatively new concept, supportive care. Previously, supportive care in cancer management used to mean rather narrowly, the use of antibiotics, blood transfusions and other medical interventions to support patients who were receiving intensive anti-cancer therapies. Latterly, supportive care in cancer and other life-limiting diseases has been seen as a comprehensive way of supporting patients and their immediate carers to cope with the screening, investigation, diagnosis, early curative or radical treatments (if feasible) and also the palliative therapies, which tend to be offered later as disease advances (Ahmedzai and Walsh 2000). In this chapter we will adopt this broader vision of comprehensive supportive care to illustrate the role of quality measures *at all stages* of the patient's journey.

In the absence of central policy on comprehensive measurement of quality of palliative care services, not surprisingly several different approaches have developed in the last 10–15 years. The measures range from specific clinical audit items, for example, symptom control, psychological support and bereavement services, to whole service accreditation. Within the past 5 years, quality tools have veered predominantly towards outcome measures, although the Donabedian criteria of structure, process and outcome are still retained within some.

Another recent UK Government initiative in this field has been the introduction of the clinical governance agenda in healthcare services. Clinical governance is basically a new way of encapsulating earlier concepts of quality assurance, risk management and audit. It uses terms such as clinical effectiveness, which is very central to current thinking on the importance of evidence-based healthcare. Thus it has been claimed that the measurement of clinical effectiveness in palliative care 'allows the evaluation and development of effective and efficacious palliative care teams' (Hearn and Higginson, 1997). Clinical governance tries to ensure that assessment-of-care outcomes form part of the compliance with national, commissioner and local provider standards of quality of care and service.

Theoretical considerations on measuring quality

In most of the tools used to assess quality in palliative care, the views of consumers of services, patients and carers are directly elicited since 'patients are usually considered to be the best judges of the symptoms they experience' (Bruera and MacDonald 1993). As exemplified above in the clinical trial comparing two analgesics, it is clear that patients themselves are also the best judge of their quality of life, even when symptom changes are apparent to clinicians. But what happens when patients are not able to share their views on symptoms and other quality-of-life dimensions? In palliative care, this is not uncommon, particularly as the patient becomes progressively weaker and less able to communicate by completing questionnaires or taking part in interviews. As discussed above, this is when it is legitimate, indeed essential, to use 'proxies' for the patients' views. The best proxy is a close family member or informal carer, preferably one who has been with the patient before the current illness as well as through the recent treatments.

Patients' views on the investigations and treatments they are prepared to undergo probably change as the disease progresses, and they may adapt to symptoms that limit their mobility or general functioning. Thus what seemed like a high level of symptom burden, for example, breathlessness from a lung cancer, at the onset of an illness, may become paradoxically less of a problem as the patient learns to avoid strenuous activities such as climbing stairs. The potential for the symptom to cause distress is still there, but the opportunities for invoking it are reduced. Furthermore, patients may become accustomed to the fear that symptoms such as breathlessness first convey and so may score it lower in a questionnaire or if asked verbally, although objectively there is still the same (or worse) degree of impairment. This tendency to adapt to the symptom is known to psychologists as 'response shift'. In such circumstances, professionals who see the patient intermittently and ask about current problems may under-score or even miss the underlying (potential) symptom, whereas a carer who has lived with the patient over the preceding weeks and months will be more likely to report their true level of distress.

A brief history of quality measures

There have been several palliative care quality assurance measures produced for use in specific areas of service (community, hospices and acute hospitals). The STAS was developed in the early 1990s (Higginson 1993) to address the work of community support teams. In its original form, it asked the team members to make judgements about the patients' and carers' experience. STAS has been used in a variety of palliative care service settings internationally.

For hospital-based or hospice services, the Edmonton Symptom Assessment System (ESAS), was produced in Canada by Bruera and colleagues (Bruera and MacDonald 1993) and is based on a series of visual analogue scales (VAS), which are completed several times a day at the bedside; for very ill patients such methods may prove problematic. The Palliative Care Assessment (PACA) tool (Ellershaw *et al.* 1995) was developed in the UK to measure the effectiveness (outcome) of interventions by the specialist hospital team. For both of these measures, staff as proxies may record changes in symptoms based on direct bedside consultations with patients, even if the latter cannot complete questionnaires themselves.

In the hospice setting, the Trent Hospice Audit Group (THAG) was formed in 1990 and pursued an approach based more in quality-of-care assessment rather than quality-of-life measurement. It first published a set of *Palliative Care Core Standards* in 1993 and then a revised second edition 5 years later (Ahmedzai *et al.* 1998). The THAG measures for these standards include items that are rated by professionals, but they also have both patient and carer interview schedules in which they are asked to identify key symptoms that are of relevance to the patient.

More recently the POS has been developed using data from a review of other outcome measures used, or proposed for use, in evaluating the palliative care of patients with advanced cancer (Hearn and Higginson, 1999). It has been designed for use in a variety of palliative care settings. There is both a staff-completed version of the questionnaire and a patient-completed version for those able to fill in the form.

Quality-of-life measures for patients undergoing clinical trials began development, as mentioned above, in Europe in the late 1980s. By 1993 Aaronson *et al.* reported on the EORTC QLQ-C30 core questionnaire for cancer patients (Aaronson *et al.* 1993). In the USA, a parallel line of research has led to the Functional Assessment of Cancer Therapy (FACT) set of scales, all of which, like the EORTC questionnaires, are designed for patients themselves to complete (Cella *et al.* 1993). Studies and wide experience have shown that they may be used as interview schedules, and they may also be completed by proxies such as staff and carers (Sneeuw *et al.* 2001).

There has been an important move towards measures that allow the patient or carer to nominate issues that are of importance to them, rather than respond to items that have been chosen by researchers. Thus, the Schedule for the Evaluation of Individual Quality of Life (SEIQoL) aims to '[give] an individual the opportunity to identify those factors that are important to him or her and to indicate the relative importance of each to overall QOL' (McGee *et al.* 1991). The McGill Quality of Life Questionnaire (MQOL) (Cohen *et al.* 1995) was designed to measure overall quality of life in people with a life-threatening illness and to indicate the areas in which the patient is doing well or poorly; it is a hybrid measure as it contains both standardized questions and areas in which patients may nominate symptoms that are important for them.

Concentrating entirely on proxies, views of bereaved carers on the quality of end-of-life care and services provided are captured in the Views of Informal Carers—Evaluation of Services (VOICES) (Addington-Hall and McPherson 2001). This is a continuation of methods originally developed in the 1960s, which were used in the large-scale Regional Study of Care of the Dying (Addington-Hall and McCarthy 1995).

Two UK developments focus on organizational audit and accreditation. First, Health Quality Service (HQS) developed from a King's Fund project in 1989, through the King's Fund Organizational Audit (from 1990 to 1993) and into an Accreditation UK Programme in 1997 covering a range of healthcare sectors (Health Quality Service 1999). The launch of the generic HQS in 1998 was followed by the development of new accreditation programme standards, including specialist palliative care services. Second, Quality by Peer Review (QPR) began as the Yorkshire Peer Review Project in 1996, involving hospices within that region (unpublished communication). It is a modular, organizational audit programme. Both of these programmes differ from most of the ones described above, in that they charge significant fees for participants and are thus more likely to be of interest to large organizations.

Current methods of assuring quality

The quality measures introduced above are now described in more detail with respect to their method of development, whether users were involved in the generation of the tools and their scope and relevance to palliative care. These and other aspects of their use, for example, whether they require registration or fees, are displayed in Table 4.1. The first column gives the name of the instrument.

How were the tools that are featured in Table 4.1 chosen? Three main criteria were used in their selection: first, they had to have at least one major publication in the palliative care field; second, they had to incorporate either a quality-of-care or a quality-of-life evaluation, or preferably both; and third, they should be feasible and practical to use in modern palliative care services. Even with these criteria, there are large differences between the measures. They fall into three broad groups (although some instruments may be counted in more than one category). These are 'clinical', 'quality of life' and 'organizational'. The category for each instrument is shown in the second column. By 'clinical', we mean measures that focus primarily on medical and to a lesser extent on nursing processes: symptom control, psychological problems and other aspects of patients' and carers' lives that are routinely assessed and acted on by palliative care teams. 'Quality of life' measures are separated because they were devised more as research tools, rather than everyday clinical instruments; however, at least one of them (the EORTC QLQ-C30) can be used in clinical settings. The 'organizational' measures are largely concerned with evaluating the structure and process of how teams and provider organizations such as hospices and hospitals offer their services. They are more concerned with quality-of-care process than outcome measures, as described above. Even within this last group, there are hybrid tools such as the THAG patient and carer interview schedules, which measure users' own symptom-oriented outcomes, as well as satisfaction with aspects of the quality of care.

The third column contains summary information about the contents of each measure: the number of items or questions and which areas or domains are covered. Column four indicates whether the measure has been published with its full criteria. It can be seen that the answer is positive for all but the QPR organizational audit system. In the fifth column we have indicated in which healthcare setting the measure was originally developed. The range includes community, hospices, other specialist palliative care units and acute hospitals.

A key criterion for describing these measures in Table 4.1 is the sixth column, in which we have tried to identify whether users themselves were involved in the development of the instrument. In some cases we have been unable, both from the published literature and from the authors, to determine this adequately. In other cases the literature informed us in some detail of how users can be incorporated in the design and testing of the instruments. For example, the EORTC Quality of Life Group has published strict guidelines on developing new modules for use in specific cancers alongside the 'core questionnaire' or QLQ-C30. These guidelines plainly state how groups of cancer patients in different clinical settings are interviewed and asked first of all to raise issues that they think are important and later to comment on and, in effect, criticize the draft questionnaires during their development. In fact, the core questionnaire itself, which was validated in extensive clinical trials involving over 500 patients and published in 1993, was not subject to this degree of user interaction in its early stages of development. On the other hand, the VOICES postal questionnaire for exploring the retrospective views of bereaved carers has explicitly involved palliative care users in the early piloting of the instrument, and in the critique and modifications that led to the latest version in 2002.

Column seven indicates in which settings the instrument, once developed, has been used or has the potential of being used. The next column shows who is meant to complete the measure. The default position is the user, and we indicate whether proxies can also be used and whether these can be carers or professional staff. The final column states whether registration with the authors is required to use the measure and also whether currently a fee is charged.

The data in Table 4.1 has been extracted from the literature and also from helpful correspondence with many of the original authors. We believe the information is accurate and up to date, but the reader should be aware that some of the tools are still in development and the properties in some of the columns may therefore change.

Analysis of the current situation

Although impressive in terms of the scope of quality-of-care and quality-of-life measurement in palliative care, a careful examination of Table 4.1 shows that there is no leading instrument, no 'gold standard' that gives the 'truest' picture. Indeed, we believe there never can be a gold standard, because to capture all possible elements of quality of care and quality of life, in all settings, with respect to patients, carers and staff, would require a very unwieldy instrument. Rather, it is helpful to view the present range of measures as options for clinicians, managers and researchers to consider and possibly combine, to obtain the most comprehensive and feasible evaluation of a particular service or intervention.

What are the limitations of the current methods? There are two main problem areas that need to be addressed in the next few years. First, the ways that users and carers are involved in the generation of issues and how these are then incorporated into a working measure, need to be improved and standardized. Some instruments have used focus groups, others individual interviews, others postal surveys. Of course it may be necessary to use different methods for specific situations. However, it would be helpful if a consensus could be reached, which should itself naturally include the views of service users, about the minimum level of user consultation and the best method to use for each clinical application. We would suggest that such a consensus could be reached by a series of workshops in which past and future instrument developers could interact with users and their representatives, to develop consensus views, based wherever possible on the literature and published evidence, and practical guidelines.

The second area for improvement is the way that users and carers are approached to provide data on quality of care and quality of life. At present data gathering is *ad hoc* and usually related to local timetables for audit and accreditation. When these audits occur, they are usually at the instruction of management and clinicians are asked to work with audit staff to produce findings and conclusions. Consultation with users about the process of conducting the audit is not often high on the agenda, as deadlines are tight and the infrastructure may not be present whereby appropriate user views can be obtained. When individual patients and carers are identified as sources of information for quality of care (for example, satisfaction survey) or quality-of-life interviews or questionnaires, the method of choosing subjects is not usually rigorous. Often a convenience sample is taken, but this may be biased in terms of the type and fitness of users, for example, very ill, uncommunicative or non-English speaking patients could be excluded. Ideally there should be guidelines about how subjects are to be identified, approached, consented and recruited into any study—whether this is for research or a local satisfaction survey. In the absence of these, it is useful to take advice from local academic centres and most large hospitals now have audit and quality assurance committees who are able to help with these choices.

View to the future

Perhaps the most challenging issue in the area of quality measurement is how, and when, to feedback the results of such surveys to the users and their groups. It is possible to argue that individuals who take part in quality assurance exercises have a right to receive feedback, on their own personal results and also the grouped results from their clinic, hospice or hospital.

This is especially true if the exercise is clearly not a research project, where rules of confidentiality and data integrity make it impossible to feedback results 'live' during the study. Many patients in palliative care quality assurance projects may not live for more than a few weeks and cannot wait for published overall results. We would argue that it is courteous and ethically sound to allow users, if they wish, to gain early feedback on their own results and also the anonymized results from the local service. Research at the Department of Oncology in Leeds has shown that patients can complete the EORTC QLQ-C30 on a touch-screen computer while waiting to see the oncologist and can get instant feedback on their scores for today (Velikova *et al.* 1999). Their doctors have access to previous scores, so these can be discussed with patients who can see instantly which elements of their quality of life are improving, staying the same or getting worse. Of course the patients 'privately' knew this, as it is merely a quantitative record of their experience, but the act of sharing this detailed form of history has the potential to enhance positively the rapport between doctor and patient.

We believe that there is a great opportunity for palliative care to develop ways of sharing quality-of-care and quality-of-life data between users and carers and users and staff, to enhance communication and understanding. This would be especially helpful as new groups of patients come within the scope of palliative care: those with non-cancer diagnoses, learning disabilities and minority ethnic backgrounds. There will need to be new ways of communicating with such diverse groups, and standardized quality measures with accessible results forms can be part of this.

As societies become enriched with greater cultural diversity, there is an increasing problem of how to capture that richness in quality assurance programmes. Cross-cultural comparisons are inevitable, especially if we wish to ensure that minority groups are not being disadvantaged or somehow are not benefiting from a palliative care service. However, there are great methodological and semantic challenges for those who seek to hear these diverse voices in our society. The WHO programme for measuring quality of life across the world has identified the problems: 'The way in which people define quality of life appears to vary significantly across cultures (i.e. how people in a given setting define a 'good life'), as do the factors that affect quality of life (i.e. access to and availability of health care, socioeconomic factors, etc.).' (Kuyken *et al.* 1994).

We believe that ultimately, more frequent and rigorous testing of the quality of care and the quality of life of our patients can allow palliative care services to become more user focused, responsive and humane.

References

Aaronson NK, Bullinger M, Ahmedzai S (1988). A modular approach to quality of life assessment in cancer clinical trials. *Recent Results Cancer Research*, 111: 231–49.

Aaronson NK, Ahmedzai S, Bergman B, Bullinger M *et al.* (1993). The European Organisation for Research and Treatment of Cancer QLQ-C30: A quality of life instrument for use in international clinical trials in oncology. *Journal of the National Cancer Institute*, 85: 365–75.

Addington-Hall J, McCarthy M (1995). Dying from cancer: results of a national population-based investigation. *Palliative Medicine*, 9: 295–305.

Addington-Hall J, McPherson C (2001). After-death interviews with surrogates/ bereaved family members: some issues of validity. *Journal of Pain and Symptom Management*, 22: 784–90.

Ahmedzai S, Brooks D (1997). Transdermal fentanyl versus sustained-release oral morphine in cancer pain: preference, efficacy, and quality of life. *Journal of Pain and Symptom Management*, 13: 254–61.

Ahmedzai SH, Walsh TD (2000). Palliative medicine and modern cancer care. *Seminars in Oncology*, 27: 1–6.

Ahmedzai S, Morton A, Reid JT, Stevenson RD (1988). Quality of death from lung cancer: patients' reports and relatives' retrospective opinions. In Watson M, Greer S, Thomas C (ed.), *Psychosocial Oncology*, pp. 187–92. Oxford: Pergamon Press.

Ahmedzai SH, Hunt J, Keeley VL (1998). *Trent Hospice Audit Group. Palliative Care Core Standards: A Multidisciplinary Approach.* Second Edition. Sheffield: University of Sheffield Press.

Bruera E, MacDonald N (1993). Audit methods: The Edmonton Symptom Assessment System. In Higginson I (ed.), *Clinical Audit in Palliative Care*, pp. 61–77. Oxford: Radcliffe Medical Press.

Calman KC, Hine D (1995). *A Policy Framework for Commissioning Cancer Services.* London: Department of Health.

Cella DF, Tulsky DS, Gray G (1993). The Functional Assessment of Cancer Therapy (FACT) Sale: development and validation of the general measure. *Journal of Clinical Oncology*, 11: 572–9.

Cohen SR, Mount BM, Strobel MG, Bui F (1995). The McGill Quality of Life Questionnaire: a measure of quality of life appropriate for people with advanced disease. A preliminary study of validity and acceptability. *Palliative Medicine*, 9: 207–19.

Department of Health (2000). *The NHS Cancer Plan.* London: Department of Health.

Donabedian A (1980). *Explorations in Quality Assessment and Monitoring: The Definition of Quality and Approaches to its Assessment*, Vol. 1. Ann Arbour, Michigan: Health Administration Press.

Ellershaw JE, Peat SJ, Boys LC (1995). Assessing the effectiveness of a hospital palliative care team. *Palliative Medicine*, 9: 145–52.

Gelber S, Gelber RD, Cole BF, Goldhirsh A (1998). Using the Q-TWiST method for treatment comparisons in clinical trials. In Staquet MJ, Hays RD, Fayers PM (ed.), *Quality of Life Assessment in Clinical Trials*, pp. 281–96. Oxford: Oxfrod University Press.

Health Quality Service (1999). *Standards Framework for Hospice Services*. First Edition. London: Health Quality Service.

Hearn J, Higginson I (1997). Outcome measures in palliative care for advanced cancer patients: a review. *Journal of Public Health Medicine*, 19: 193–9.

Hearn J, Higginson I (1999). Development and validation of a core outcome measure for palliative care: the palliative care outcome scale. *Quality in Health Care*, 8: 219–27.

Heaven CM, McGuire P (1997). Disclosure of concerns by hospice patients and their identification by nurses. *Palliative Medicine*, 11: 283–90.

Higginson I (1993). Audit methods: a community schedule. In Higginson I (ed.), *Clinical Audit in Palliative Care*, pp. 34–47. Oxford: Radcliffe Medical Press.

Karnofsky DA, Burchenal JH (1949). The clinical evaluation of chemotherapeutic agents in cancer. In Macleod CM (ed.), *Evaluation of Chemotherapeutic Agents*, p. 191. New York: Columbia University Press.

Kuyken W, Orley J, Hudelson P, Sartorius N (1994). Quality of life assessment across cultures. *International Journal of Mental Health*, 23(2): 5–27.

McGee H, O'Boyle CA, Hickey A, O'Malley K, Joyce CRB (1991). Assessing the quality of life of the individual: SEIQoL with a healthy and a gastroenterology unit population. *Psychological Medicine*, 21: 749–59.

Morita T, Adachi I (2002). Satisfaction with rehydration therapy for terminally ill cancer patients: concept construction, scale development, and identification of contributing factors. *Support Care Cancer*, 10: 44–50.

O'Brien J, Francis A (1988). The use next-of-kin to estimate pain in cancer outpatients. *Pain*, 35: 171–8.

Sneeuw KW, Albertsen PC, Aaronson NK (2001). Comparison of patient and spouse assessments of health related quality of life in men with metastatic prostate cancer. *Jounal of Urology* 165: 478–82.

Sulmasy DP, McIlvane JM, Pasley PM, Rahn M (2002). A scale for measuring patient perceptions of the quality of end-of-life care and satisfaction with treatment: the reliability and validity of QUEST. *Journal of Pain and Symptom Management*, 23: 458–70.

Thompson G, McClement S (2002). Defining and determining quality in end-of-life care. *International Journal of Palliative Nursing*, 8: 288–93.

Twycross RG (1987) Quality before quantity—a note of caution. *Palliative Medicine*, 1: 65–72.

Velikova G, Wright EP, Smith AB, Cull A, Gould A, Forman D, Perren T, Stead M, Brown J, Selby PJ (1999). Automated collection of quality-of-life data: a comparison of paper and computer touch-screen questionnaires. *Journal of Clinical Oncology*, 17: 998–1007.

Ware JE, Gandek B and the IQOLA Project Group (1994). The SF-36 Health Survey: development and use in mental health research and the IQOLA project. *International Journal of Mental Health*, 23: 49–73.

WHO (1990). *Cancer Pain Relief and Palliative Care*. Technical Report 804. Geneva: WHO.

5

Education in palliative care

Emma Davie and Bill Noble

Introduction

Palliative care, with its focus on patient- and family-centred care, has the potential, as much as any other specialty, to embrace the voice of service users as a resource for students.

Clinicians understand the value of learning from their patients. It is rarely possible to emerge from a clinical encounter without learning a lesson for future practice. The challenge is to carry this experience over into our educational endeavours. We must take our patients' agenda seriously when training the next generation of our colleagues.

Respect for our patients' predicament and the need for an uncluttered therapeutic relationship, make the involvement of patients in educational activity problematic. The hospice movement and palliative medicine appeared too late to be associated with body-snatchers and the worst excesses of clinical demonstrations associated with older medical schools. However there is a sensitivity about involving patients receiving palliative care in medical education usually born of an awareness of patients' limited survival and sometimes fragile coping mechanisms. In spite of this, clinicians involved in the subject have developed an interest and expertise in education disproportionate to the size of the specialty. The voluntary hospice movement has embraced nursing and medical education as a central strategy for promoting the principles of palliative care to other health workers.

Public policy in the UK concerning palliative care in medical and nursing education is a recent development. The Wilkes report (Wilkes 1980) was the first policy document to recommend the inclusion of terminal care in the undergraduate medical curriculum. In 1993, the Association for Palliative Medicine produced its Palliative Medicine Curriculum with many learning outcomes for medical students as well as those for specialists in training. None of these prescribed the involvement of users in either the design or delivery of learning in palliative care.

Within medical schools a variety of teaching methods have been developed with patients and families involved directly and indirectly through video interviews, case histories and narratives. The most recent survey of palliative care education in UK medical schools (Field and Wee in press) concluded that the subject was taught by all 24 programmes reporting. Topics covered by at least 92% of courses included attitudes towards death and dying, symptom relief in advanced terminal disease, analgesics for chronic pain, analgesics for cancer pain, communication with family members of dying patients, grief and bereavement and psychological aspects of dying.

The mean number of taught hours in palliative care was 20 in 2001 (range 6–100), compared to a mean of 6 in 1983 and 3 in 1994.

The General Medical Council's document, *Tomorrow's doctors* (General Medical Council 1993) has recommended a reduction of factual learning, a variety of teaching methods and an expansion in special study modules, which are opportunities for students to research or gain experience in specific subjects in depth. Palliative care is offered as one of these subjects by many schools. Communication skills, ethics and reflective practice are integrated throughout many curriculae and palliative care provides a useful setting for delivering this learning (Field and Wee in press).

Teaching methods increasingly include role play and hospice clinical attachments and seven schools reported that terminally ill patients routinely address the class with three facilitating one-to-one contact between students and palliative care patients.

Nurses on the other hand received rather less palliative care training in 2001, with an average of 7.8 hours (range 2 to 26 hours) on diploma courses and 12.2 hours (range 3 to 42 hours) on degree courses. Theoretical teaching predominated and tutors reported a shortage of suitably skilled staff to teach palliative care and a similar shortage of clinical placements in the subject (Lloyd-Williams and Field in press).

An example of user involvement in interprofessional learning

Although contact between students and patients receiving palliative care in the clinical context is becoming commonplace, the transition from patient to service user is beginning to be seen by students on a few courses.

This transition from passive reporter of symptoms and concerns to an agent with an agenda for influencing the characteristics of clinicians comes when patients and carers are invited to share their story with students and interpret its meaning.

In Southampton, half day interprofessional workshops in palliative care include medical, nursing, physiotherapy, occupational therapy and social work students (Wee *et al.* 2001). After some work on professional roles, small groups of students hear a family carer selected at random from the ranks of bereaved relatives or families of current patients. The aim is for students to reflect on the carer's experience and undertake specific tasks related to consideration of how different professionals deliver care within a team and how this can be improved. Carers take the opportunity to unload feelings as well as views in an environment supervised by a workshop facilitator who takes responsibility for debriefing and responding to important issues. The presence of more than one discipline in the group provides experiential learning as students support each other in eliciting the story as well as the carer whilst they give an account and offer their views on what has happened to a particular patient.

Student evaluation of the teaching is positive, they value and enjoy the opportunity to learn together. Feedback from carers indicates that they value the opportunity to present real-life experience to students. The logistics of this method of teaching are difficult but, as the authors have demonstrated, not impossible.

User involvement in a communication skills course

Final-year medical students at the University of Sheffield Medical School spend 7 weeks in general practice. During this clinical attachment, six afternoons are spent in seminars and small groups on communication. The teaching is delivered by a multi-professional group and includes

- small group work revising communication theory, discussion and role playing key issues in the general practice consultation;
- briefing and debriefing following home visits with day hospice patients or bereaved relatives where the task is to elicit their concerns;
- role play and group discussion of two bad news scenarios:
    dealing with a serious diagnosis
    dealing with sudden death;
- patient interview in general practice.

There are seven learning outcomes: key communication skills that students need to acquire and on which they are tested at the end of the module.

1. *Gaining and maintaining a rapport with the patients*
   Introduction, explanation, politeness, eye contact, appropriate body language, empathy.

2. *Helping the patient to talk*
   Use of open questions, facilitation, echoing, picking up verbal and non-verbal cues, use of silence, reflecting back.

3. *Gathering accurate information*
   Clarifying, checking out, asking for examples, exploring feelings, asking about psychological and social aspects of the problem.

4. *Maintaining a smooth flow to the consultation*
   Following the patient's agenda and cues. Listening, matching pace, not interrupting.

5. *Focusing and directing the consultation*
   Use of focused and closed questions, summarizing, giving appropriate information.

6. *Understanding the problems from the patient's perspective*
   Having a clear view of why the patient has consulted and what their beliefs, concerns and expectations are.

7. *Dealing with feelings*
   Managing the emotions of patients and yourself in a sensitive and responsible manner

The interview with bereaved carers or hospice day patients is the opportunity for pairs of medical students to hear stories that may include powerful messages for a trainee doctor. This is where service users are given an opportunity to speak directly to future clinicians.

The task for both kinds of interview is to elicit patients' serious concerns and to discuss the impact of either an illness or bereavement on their life. Students list and discuss these concerns during the session after the interview and they inform the role play held after debriefing. The group is encouraged to focus on how the concerns impact on the individual's health care. Common themes between interviews are also discussed and students are encouraged to reflect on the diversity of experience reported by the group.

Evaluation was provided by 124 students by completing a six-point scale in the academic year 1999/2000. Sixty-six per cent reported agreement that the course had improved their communication skills. Seventy per cent reported that their knowledge of communication had been broadened.

Comments included opinions that the training is useful and should appear earlier in the course.

Students undergo an assessment by objective structured clinical exam (OSCE) of two simulated patient consultation stations. In the academic year 1999/2000, all 202 students passed, one after re-sitting the OSCE. Six distinctions were awarded.

User involvement

Debriefing sessions with groups of medical students are led by a specialist registrar and the social worker. The use of facilitators with these backgrounds integrates the principles and practices of medicine and social work. It enhances the voice of the user by discussion. It demonstrates to medical students, by the style of debriefing used, that different disciplines working together can better address issues of pain and suffering in the best interests of patients and bereaved people.

A study by Wilkes (1993) quoted by Sheldon (2001) found that in a survey of hospice bereavement services the majority were run by social workers. Wilkes observes

... the main burden of organising training and of dealing with difficult selected cases is most usually seen as the responsibility of the social worker.

All Diploma in Social Work courses include as a knowledge base

... the emotional impact of traumatic events and the range of emotional and psychological reactions to loss, transition and change.
(Central Council for Education and Training in Social Work 1996).

This is cited by Oliviere (2001) who reminds us that the body, mind and spirit are

... housed in a context of family, neighbourhood, community and society ... essentially within relationships. This is social work, assessing and intervening with the patient and family and their wider connections.

Legislation since the Seebohm Report (1968) has recognized that the needs of people should be taken into account in policy making and planning. The Children Act (1989) and National Health Service and Community Care Act (1990) have emphasized this and user involvement has become an essential part of developing health and social services.

Social work clients are involved in case conferences and care plan meetings. Patients are also becoming more involved in decisions concerning their care and there is now an emphasis on all disciplines to give information in a way that increases understanding and helps users to be part of the decision-making process. Fallowfield (2001) writes

> ... there is a compelling need for training and other interventions to help communication between doctors and patients about the likely and preferred therapeutic goals and priorities of treatment.

Bereaved people as users

A number of bereaved people are identified as users within the Bereavement Service at St Lukes Hospice, where ways of support are varied to meet the whole range of needs experienced by grieving individuals. Some may attend a specific group or meeting and some may have one-to-one support. In addition to these users, bereaved people who have experienced the loss of a child or children or loss through suicide, road traffic accident, sudden death or major disaster are recruited by the social work author who draws on a background of paediatric social work, child protection, social work in a palliative care setting and also home finding and respite care for children with disabilities or short-life expectation. When appropriate, additional users are recruited by the author, through her ongoing work as a trainer for CRUSE Bereavement Care Sheffield.

Patients with a serious diagnosis are also identified by St Lukes Hospice as users. They attend day hospice and have consented to be interviewed by pairs of students. Nurses are responsible for recruitment, preparation and the debriefing of patients.

Each bereaved person and patient is unique in their experience and reactions. In serious illness grief starts at diagnosis and prognosis with all the implications and fears for the future and the death.

Different experiences of loss

In bereavement *the how, who and where* the person died and previous life experiences will affect grief. Field and James (1993) examined variations and experience of dying people according to the place of care. It is usual that everything involved in that experience will impact on the carer and affect the bereavement.

We should aim therefore to select users with a variety of different experiences of loss, who are sufficiently articulate to express their feelings and describe the effect that loss has had on their lives. From the onset users need help to acknowledge and understand that focusing back into their own experience of loss is emotionally painful, albeit normal. Users are given guidance and support in the task, which enables and strengthens them. They often comment that the whole user experience has been therapeutic.

Different loss experiences prompt wide discussion in medical student feedback and examples of different loss are set out below.

User A's father died from a brain tumor 3 weeks after the diagnosis. He had been unwell for several months. The user is a single parent and has a teenage daughter who has a congenital heart condition. Prognosis is uncertain. Discussions centre on the experience of caring for her father, the mishandling of the diagnosis and her feelings of intense anger immediately following his death. The user also discusses the fears and uncertainties of open-ended grief associated with her daughter's medical condition and short-life expectancy (Alderson 1990).

User B has experienced two losses through suicide. Issues discussed are that grief reactions are often more intense after traumatic loss, particularly feelings of anger and guilt. The user describes how following the suicides she suffered a nervous breakdown. This affected relationships within the family and resulted in divorce. This in turn affected her children. The total experience of loss affected her career, led to further professional training and a complete change in lifestyle. Students will learn how a cascade of losses can stem from traumatic bereavement and how each loss brings about change in a person's life.

User C looked after her husband throughout a long illness. Her professional skills enabled him to remain at home with the family until shortly before his death. The teenage children were well informed and involved in his care. Preservation of the patient's dignity was of paramount importance. Towards the end of the patient's life it was anticipated that the actual process of dying would be complicated. A decision was made by the patient and family that to ensure a good death he would not die at home as originally planned but in an establishment of their choosing. User C's experience was that when her husband became an in-patient the professional staff did not understand the illness and lacked the skills to keep him comfortable. The patient died in pain, fear and without dignity.

Medical students learn from User C that even when an illness is understood and well managed by carers, bereavement can become complicated if professional carers are not able to provide the expertise to ensure a good death. User C also discusses with students the differences and difficulties of coping with personal grief whilst working as a professional carer and how this experience has refashioned her thinking and changed her practice.

Several of the team of users have multiple losses, some whose partners died from cancer have the same illness. By considering the mix of experiences of each group of users allocated to students, feedback sessions become interesting and thought provoking. The different scenarios are discussed and where appropriate students reflect on theories of grief. By working in this manner medical students begin to see users in the context of family and friends and are helped to identify how the psychological and practical issues associated with death and dying impact on life.

In feedback students have the user's story to relate and this can be examined and developed further to broaden learning within the group. User A's experience of the unexpected death of her father and the trauma associated with sudden death can be compared to the experience of caring long term for a seriously ill person with all the uncertainties and swings from hope to despair and the physical and emotional exhaustion suffered by User C. The benefits and burdens of sudden death compared to that which is anticipated are examined.

Grief in children and their understanding of death are explored in the light of User C's children growing up with a terminally ill parent and User A's daughter whose life expectancy is uncertain. These topics are discussed having in mind that children vary in their intellectual, emotional and physical development and depending upon chronological age.

Discussions can be as broad or deep as contacts with patients and bereaved people allow and time permits.

From User B's experience discussions can be developed around the inquest, publicity and society's attitude to suicide and how they affect grieving. Students note that a high proportion of those who attempt suicide have suffered major changes or life events in the preceding year. They learn that bereavement itself carries a high risk of morbidity and suicide attempts may occur when the reality of the bereaved person's changed situation is realized but not adjusted to.

In looking at user experience and seeing each person as part of family and community students begin to learn that people are bound together by a common humanity.

Support of bereaved people as users

Users need to feel safe and to know that they can make contact for support or discussion at any time. A user whose friend died recently from cancer, whose brother-in-law died after a long illness and whose son-in-law drowned, needed to meet and talk at length on the anniversary of the death by drowning of her 2-year-old son in 1980. The vivid recall of her son's death had been triggered by the recent loss of her friend from cancer. This vivid recall had also happened when her son-in-law died 3 years ago.

Similarly, a further user whose son and foster child died in a house fire several years ago needed contact and support at the time of the Alderhay enquiry. On checking with the coroner she found that organs from her son had been used in research. Her grief was deep and raw and her recall detailed. She graphically described the hospital experience at the time of the deaths and how she was given no time to hold the children or 'kiss them better'. With help the user has been able to include her reaction to Alderhay into the discussions with students. The experience demonstrates to students how a person can integrate loss into their lives and move forward, building a new life around their grief (Tonkin 1996).

On average bereaved people in the role of user link with students once during the academic year. In total users are used three times before retiring. This is to ensure the task does not become a burden and that the story does not become rehearsed. Recruitment of users is ongoing.

Bereaved people are supported as users by the author on an individual basis in conjunction with peer group meetings when appropriate.

Points for further discussion

Considering user involvement allows us to interrogate the relationship between citizen and state in the context of the citizen living with a particular illness. As such it illuminates questions of meaning at the level of the individual and questions of power at the level of the state and the professions.

(Small and Rhodes 2000)

In recruiting users and taking feedback from them and from students, questions are raised that need discussion and consideration.

How should we recruit? Do we ask for volunteers or do we seek out and approach individuals who will provide the right teaching material? Do people want to participate in training, how do they feel and how do we think they feel? Preparation for the task needs to be sensitive and thorough to prevent damage to already vulnerable people.

Recruiters have a responsibility in the preparation of users and in taking feedback from them after the student contact, to reassure and affirm their worth. Work with users may also raise issues linked to their experiences that need addressing at a personal level or that may have implications on institutional policy or professional practice.

Similarly, medical students may be vulnerable because of their own life experiences or apprehensive about the task in hand and may need to have support. Should students be exposed to situations which they would prefer not to handle or can difficult and unexpected incidents be used positively as part of a learning process? Is it safer for students to be confronted by difficult situations whilst in the protected environment of medical school where there is the opportunity to examine in a training setting problems that arise rather than be over protective? It is a difficult balance.

Reflections on involving users in palliative care education

There are limitations to a users' perspective on how clinicians and health professionals should be educated. Rare conditions or health issues in which patients die quickly without much experience of 'userhood' will be under-represented within the voice of the user. Those patients who leave no-one grieving or who are surrounded only by professional carers within institutions lack advocates. Those too young to make cogent representation nevertheless have needs and their interests should be considered. These are numerically important groups, particularly when all those patients with rare conditions are considered as one group, but who gives voice to their needs as other views become stronger and more vocal groups of users gain our attention?

In education, health professionals' perception of issues important to service users may be modified by information with a public health perspective and the experience of learning medicine in the context of primary care. Learning in generic care settings allows students to identify which issues arise rarely and which are common to many categories of health service user.

An important concept for students is that of the diversity of users' needs and views. Here, reference to students' views as service users or potential users can be valuable. 'How would you want your doctor or nurse to be when they … ?' is a useful question that brings out the user in most students. Contrasting their views with those of users allows students the insight to put their own views in the context of the general public. In this way they can discover which views are almost universal, which are held by substantial proportions of users and which are idiosyncratic.

Users are finally being involved in the design of new medical courses and there is the potential for a more patient-focused agenda across many areas of health care education. However as we have described, users are an educational resource requiring care and attention. Sources of users willing to participate need to be cultivated, nurtured and not exploited beyond their capacity. Perhaps the greatest threat to the goodwill of users is now the volume of educational activity in the field. The onerous, repetitive and demanding task of simulating patients in the context of student assessment is best undertaken by actors rather than bereaved relatives or ex-patients. Performance and responses to students, above all else, need to be standardized and fair to each candidate. It is difficult for users to sustain this kind of activity dispassionately as well as maintaining enthusiasm year after year. The dangers of triggering old feelings and grief in role playing simulated patients has precluded the involvement of users in examinations where communication skills are tested.

The role of the patient in medical and nursing education could be described as a continuum from unwilling victim at one end, then fascinating example, good case and central object of study, to a consultant in the training of health professionals.

The relationship between patients, students and their teachers is potentially one of equal partnership because students and teachers need patients as much as patients need doctors, nurses and other trained health workers.

Acknowledgements

The teaching programme described at St Luke's Hospice in Sheffield was originally devised by Professor Eric Wilkes and Dr Tony Crowther and delivered by Dr Simon O'Connor. The general practice teaching in Sheffield is co-ordinated and evaluated by Dr Ivan Appelqvist. The secretarial support for this programme and report was provided by Mrs Joanne Brodie and Mrs Anita Taylor.

References

Alderson P (1990). *Choosing for Children: Parents Consent to Surgery*. Oxford University Press, Oxford.

Central Council for Education and Training in Social Work (1996). *Assuring Quality in the Diploma in Social Work—1. Rules and Requirements for the Diploma Social Work*. Second Revision. Central Council for Education and Training in Social Work, London.

Fallowfield L (2001). Participation of patients in decisions about treatment for cancer. Desire for information is not the same as a desire to participate in decision making. *British Medical Journal* 323(7322):1144.

Field D and James N (1993). *Where and How People Die. Death, Dying and Bereavement. Future Issues in Policy and Practice.* Open University Press, Buckingham.

Field D and Wee B (in press). Preparation for palliative care: Teaching about death, dying and bereavement in UK medical schools 2000–2001. *Medical Education.*

General Medical Council (1993). *Tomorrow's Doctors: Recommendations on Undergraduate Medical Education.* GMC, London.

Lloyd-Williams M and Field D (in press). What do undergraduate nurses learn about palliative care during their training? *Nurse Education Today.*

National Health Service and Community Care Act (1990). The Stationery Office, London.

Oliviere D (2001). The social worker in palliative care—the eccentric role. *Progress in Palliative Care* 9:237–41.

Seebohm Report (1968). *Report by the Committee on Local Authority and Allied Social Service.* HMSO, London.

Sheldon F (2001). Social work in palliative care: counselling and communicating. *Progress in Palliative Care* 9:242–3.

Small N and Rhodes P (2000). *Too Ill to Talk? User Involvement in Palliative Care.* Routledge, London.

The Children Act (1989). The Stationery Office, London.

Tonkin L (1996). Growing around grief, another way of looking at grief and recovery. *Bereavement Care* 15:10.

Wee B, Hillier R, Coles C, Mountford B, Sheldon F and Turner P (2001). Palliative care: a suitable setting for undergraduate interprofessional education. *Palliative Medicine* 15:487–92.

Wilkes E (Chair, Standing Medical Advisory Committee) (1980). *Terminal Care: Report of Working Group.* HMSO, London.

Wilkes E (1993). Characteristics of hospice bereavement services. *Journal Cancer Care* 2:183–9.

6

Cultural difference and palliative care

Juan M. Núñez Olarte

Introduction

Culture could be defined as 'that complex whole which includes knowledge, belief, art, morals, law, custom and any other capabilities and habits acquired by man as a member of society' (Tylor 1971). The influence of culture is very pervasive. It is not restricted to religious rituals and can be detected in several aspects of advanced cancer care. Other terms that have been used instead of culture in the palliative care setting are nationality, ethnicity, race, faith and religion.

The concept of 'care' is strongly related to the cultural and historical roots of a society. There is no such thing as a non-temporal and universal idea of care. Caring is different depending on the context. Today there is a general consensus in our societies that a new philosophy of caring is needed, underpinning the emergence of 'palliative care'. But this general philosophy is also differently interpreted and applied in diverse socio-cultural contexts. Therefore there are distinct organizational models of delivering end-of-life care around the world (Núñez Olarte and Gracia Guillén 2001; Clark *et al.* 2000).

Existing issues in end-of-life care related to culture

Traditionally culture has been associated with some issues considered to be relevant in palliative care (Neuberger 1998; Oliviere 1999; Latimer 2000):

◆ rituals of dying and death;

◆ patterns of grieving and the grieving process itself;

- gender roles and family systems;
- emotional expression and sharing;
- dietary requirements and use of alternative therapies;
- beliefs about causation of illness.

New issues in palliative care related to culture

There are several 'new' issues emerging in the care of terminally ill patients that are related to culture (Núñez Olarte and Gracia Guillén 2001; Núñez Olarte 1999; Bates *et al.* 1993; Núñez Olarte *et al.* 2000):

- terminal sedation versus euthanasia;
- last 48 hours of life versus traditions of *agonía* (a unique Hispanic cultural way of confronting the state prior to death where a slow slipping away of the senses is expected);
- definition of 'terminality';
- hospice versus non-hospice traditions;
- external versus internal *locus of control* and acceptance of death;
- perceived value of disclosure and cognition;
- opioid and psychotropic prescription;
- communication, diagnosis disclosure, truth-telling.

Influence of culture on patients' perception of pain and treatment

Certain cultural traditions hold the view that reality is not completely controllable, as humans can control only certain aspects of their environment and life. North American researchers tend to see this as a passive and pessimistic attitude, whereas researchers from other cultures view it as realistic. The psychological construct known as locus of control (LOC) style helps to frame this difference. When viewed as ideal types, an internal LOC style involves a reported perception that life events and circumstances are the result of one's own actions, whereas an external LOC style includes the perception that they are beyond one's own control, in the hands of fate, chance or other people (Bates *et al.* 1993).

Research has shown that cultural background is significantly related not only to differences in response to chronic pain, but also to differences in reported pain perception in laboratory pain studies (Edwards *et al.* 2001).

Patients from minority ethnic communities in any society have been found to receive inadequate pain treatment and better assessment is certainly needed (Cleeland *et al.* 1997). Nevertheless stereotyping patients from certain ethnic groups is inappropriate as there are always significant interindividual variations.

Culture and 'quality of death'

Several of the new issues mentioned above are connected in a wider sense. In spite of the sincere efforts of health professionals world-wide to avoid 'generalizing' the experience of dying patients under their care, we nevertheless have to use theoretical constructs (stages, phases and so on) to help us conceptualize important life transitions. Inevitably these constructs convey the message that there is some 'right way' or ways of dying and that these right ways to die involve the thinking, feeling, saying and doing of certain things and the avoidance of other thoughts and behaviours.

This tendency towards the idea that there is a 'thanatologically correct' way to die has been constantly challenged. Roy, speaking from the ethical perspective, asks 'Who really knows how to die?' (Roy 2000). Sandman, speaking from the philosophical perspective, asks 'What is a good death?' (Dekkers *et al.* 2002). From a Buddhist perspective, whether the person openly accepts death or not does not matter (Bainbridge and Baines 2001). Recent qualitative research with an in-depth ethnographic technique of interviewing has disclosed an amazing wealth of data in the biographical narratives of dying patients (Yedidia and MacGregor 2001). The diversity of ways of relating to the prospect of dying in this study might suggest that there is no way of finding 'common ground' within everybody's rich trajectory or life story. The 'uniqueness' of the dying experience in any given human being will preclude any attempt to compare the experience. On the other hand the authors concluded that outlooks on dying among the American patients interviewed for this study were thoroughly grounded in the frames of reference that gave meaning and consistency to other major events in their lives. Culture is certainly one of these 'frames of reference'.

The recent debate in Western society on euthanasia and physician-assisted suicide (PAS) and the need to audit the care provided at the end of life by specialist palliative care services has triggered very interesting quantitative research. Although this research is not without important limitations, it provides very interesting insights into 'quality of care at end of life', a concept that could be exchanged with that of 'quality of death'. What is being evaluated in these studies is important considerations at the end of life, simultaneously encompassing attributes of a 'good death'.

An attempt to summarize and compare the data from three of these studies (Bayés *et al.* 2000; Steinhauser *et al.* 2000; Singer *et al.* 1999) is presented in Table 6.1. Notwithstanding small differences in methodology, the fact remains that the relative importance ascribed by health professionals involved in palliative care to the different components of a 'good death' in the Spanish study (Bayés *et al.* 2000) is strikingly different to the American one (Steinhauser *et al.* 2000). The Spanish professionals give highest priority to family interaction (having relatives around and being able to communicate with them) and lowest to being at peace with God. They also seem to be more concerned about the emotional and financial impact on their families than their American counterparts. Explaining the differences by suggesting that Spanish professionals have better access to pain control than their American colleagues seems too simplistic. Possibly the difference lies in the societies and their culture. Also within the American study (Steinhauser *et al.* 2000) significant differences are found related to ethnic backgrounds and religiosity. African American and other non-white ethnic groups were significantly more likely than white participants to agree with the importance of using all available treatments. Participants who considered faith or spirituality unimportant were significantly more likely to wish to control the time and place of their death than were those who considered it very important.

The family acts as a focal social unit in much of southern Europe at the interface between the patient and health-care services. It is common practice in these countries to inform a member of the patient's family about the diagnosis, allowing the family to determine what information the patient receives. Evidence has been provided about this key role performed by families thanks to qualitative and quantitative research performed by psychologists (Meseguer *et al.* 1995) and social assistants (Cabrera Bermudes *et al.* 2000; F. Ruiz *et al.*, Palliative Care Unit support groups for relatives, unpublished communication). Families in far-east Asia also play this key role looking after their dying members within their own cultural ways (Maddocks 2000). In Pune (India) relatives are seen as a precious resource and one of the criteria for admission to palliative care services is that a relative accompanies the patient and is willing to be taught how to give drugs or naso-gastric or gastrostomy feeds or manage fungating wounds (Burn 2001). A strong, supportive family network and withholding of information by relatives to patients seems also to be characteristic of non-white, especially Asian, minorities in the UK (Karim *et al.* 2000).

Table 6.1 Important considerations at the end of life or attributes of a 'good death' of Spanish health professionals (Bayés et al. 2000), American health professionals and patients (Steinhauser et al. 2000) and Canadian patients (Singer et al. 1999)

Important considerations	Rank order health professionals (Bayés et al. 2000)	Rank order health professionals (Steinhauser et al. 2000)	Rank order patients (Steinhauser et al. 2000)	Rank order patients (Singer et al. 1999)
Family interaction	1	2	3	3
Freedom from pain	3	1	1	5
Avoid prolongation	6			1
At peace with God	11	3	2	
Feel life was meaningful	2	4	7	
Feeling of control	5			2
Avoid burden on family—finances	4	8–9	6	4
Resolve conflicts	7	6	8	
Die at home	10	8–9	9	
Treatment choices followed		5	5	
Mentally aware		7	4	

It is easy to perceive these family models as old fashioned and certainly doomed in a rapidly changing globalized world. Furthermore, some may think that their influence is negative in the overall 'quality of death' of the dying patient. On the other hand we have recent evidence that these family systems are not so negative. Of a sample of 513 American elderly patients, 70.8% preferred to have their family and physician make resuscitation decisions for them. In the same study of a sample of 646 seriously ill adult patients, 78% preferred to have their family and physician decide on resuscitation (Puchalski *et al.* 2000). In another American study mentioned above (Steinhauser *et al.* 2000) the highest degree of consensus between the different groups was reached precisely on the importance of naming someone to make decisions (Steinhauser *et al.* 2001). Perhaps as the authors of one of the studies (Puchalski *et al.* 2000) conclude, patients' preferences are best understood not in isolation, but within a broader context of patient values, cultural traditions, spiritual beliefs and social relationships.

Euthanasia and physician-assisted suicide versus terminal sedation

What is the acceptability of euthanasia and PAS in different cultural settings? Some studies have attempted to address the issue by asking terminally ill patients themselves. In a seminal study (Emanuel *et al.* 2000) with an American sample of 988 terminally ill patients the investigators found that African Americans and religious individuals are more likely to oppose euthanasia or PAS. Another study with an American sample of 92 terminally ill cancer patients (Rosenfeld *et al.* 2000) also found significant differences across ethnic groups, with white patients endorsing greater numbers of items in a self-report measure of desire for death than African American and Hispanic patients. Interestingly there is also evidence of the influence of ethnicity on physician attitudes towards patient autonomy, advance care directives and preferences for end-of-life decision making (Blackhall *et al.* 1995; Mebane *et al.* 1999).

Culture can also be detected behind the low support for euthanasia and PAS in Italian general practitioners, with religious beliefs, specifically a Catholic affiliation, having a strong influence (Grassi *et al.* 1999). At the other end of the spectrum, after adjusting for potential confounding factors, nationality has remained the most important predictor of physicians' attitudes and practices in neonatal end-of-life decision making in 10 European countries (Rebagliato *et al.* 2000). Finally euthanasia was not considered an option for Muslim groups in a recent South African study (Hosking *et al.* 2000).

In some countries the debate on euthanasia and PAS is shifting towards or including the debate on terminal sedation and there is a growing consensus about the perception that the ethical dilemma nowadays is not 'euthanasia yes or no' but 'sedation when and how' (Núñez Olarte and Gracia Guillén 2001). Terminal sedation has been defined as

> the deliberate administration of drugs in order to induce a sufficiently profound and presumably irreversible reduction of consciousness in a patient close to death, with the intention of alleviating refractory physical and/or psychological suffering and with the explicit, implicit or delegated consent of the patient.
>
> (Porta *et al.* 1999).

Terminal sedation is usually considered in the setting of patients with a very limited life expectancy—either days or weeks. In Spanish culture the phases of *agonía* and *preagonía* approximately match this limited prognosis of days or weeks and are therefore considered an acceptable time frame to consider terminal sedation (Couceiro and Núñez Olarte 2001). The slow slipping away of the senses the Spanish call *agonía* (Clark 2001) is strikingly similar to the Buddhist approach to the last days of life (Bainbridge and Baines 2001).

The issue of psychological distress or suffering as a reason for terminal sedation is a recent arrival in the literature. The studies that accept this indication have all been performed outside the Anglo-Saxon North-American cultural environment: Spain, four studies (Porta Sales *et al.* 1999; Viguria Arrieta *et al.* 1999; Fainsinger *et al.* 2000; Pascual and Gisbert 2000); Italy, one study (Peruselli *et al.* 1999); Japan, one study (Morita 1999); and the UK, one study (Stone *et al.* 1997). On the other hand some authors suggest that terminal sedation might not be acceptable within certain Jewish (Azoulay *et al.* 2000) and Muslim traditions (Hosking *et al.* 2000).

Cultural factors have an impact on the decision about and the social acceptability of sedation for psychological suffering, with clear links to the tradition of *agonía* in Hispanic societies (Fainsinger *et al.* 2000; Núñez Olarte and Gracia Guillén 2001). A recent comparative study has shown that Spanish terminal patients and their families ascribe less relevance to the preservation of cognition and diagnosis disclosure than their counterparts in Canada (Núñez Olarte *et al.* 2000).

Diagnosis disclosure

The last decade has witnessed a transition in health professionals in the UK and USA from 'full open disclosure' to 'conditional disclosure' of terminal diagnosis and prognosis when confronting dying patients (Field and

Copp 1999). Simultaneously research in countries such as Spain (Centeno Cortés and Núñez Olarte 1994; Centeno Cortés and Núñez Olarte 1998), Italy (Grassi *et al.* 2000; Tamburini *et al.* 2000), Japan (Charlton *et al.* 1995; Seo *et al.* 2000), Greece (Mystakidou *et al.* 1996), Portugal (Pimentel *et al.* 2000; Gonçalves and Castro 2001), Israel (Sapir *et al.* 2000), France (Valera and Aubry 2000), Colombia (Fonnegra de Jaramillo 1992), the Philippines (Ngelangel *et al.* 1996), Taiwan (Lin 1999) and Hong-Kong (Fielding *et al.* 1998) has prompted a review of the long-held assumption that diagnosis disclosure is always in the best interest of the patient. There are different cultural reasons in every country or region that support its degree of commitment to 'truth-telling', as studies in minorities within the USA (Blackhall *et al.* 1995; Berger *et al.* 2000; Curtis *et al.* 2000), the UK (Koffman *et al.* 1999; Spruyt 1999) and Australia (Chan and Woodruff 1992) clearly indicate. Some studies bear witness to the difficulties even 'majority culture' terminally ill patients in the USA have in discussing their personal fears (Steinhauser *et al.* 2001).

With the available evidence it is difficult to support the 'open awareness' approach that was so prevalent in the early literature in palliative care. Some recent studies are starting to tackle the difficult issue of communication styles and their impact in the care of advanced cancer patients (Tamburini *et al.* 2000; Bruera *et al.* 2000*a*; Friedrichsen *et al.* 2000). Some authors are suggesting the use of advanced directives in communication given the perceived complexities (Hammes 2000; Fetters and Masuda 2000; Seo *et al.* 2000). However the cultural failure of advanced directives is already an established fact (Solomon 2000). Furthermore attitudes towards communication amongst physicians seem to be culturally driven (Bruera *et al.* 2000*b*). There are even deeper levels of analysis, some suggesting that breaking bad news is part of a 'ritual' in the process of adapting to terminal disease (Lynn 2000) and others attempting to connect communication with death acceptance (see Table 6.2).

The cultural traditions of non-disclosure stand in contrast to the emerging ethic of autonomy. Labelling these traditions as 'right' or 'wrong' is simplistic. There are already indications mentioned above that the two approaches have more in common than expected. It is exactly in the confrontation that new, fruitful perspectives can be found (Janssens *et al.* 2001).

Meeting diverse needs in a multi-cultural society

Some useful pointers may be provided by experience and research.

◆ Evaluate the preference in communication and decision-making style of your patient and their family.

Table 6.2 Preliminary proposal of a theoretical construct that might explain perceived differences in acceptance of death between patients and families in Spain and the USA

Differences	Patient	Family
Cognitive acceptance of death	**No (denial)**/*Yes*	**Yes**/*Yes*
Emotional acceptance of death	**Yes**/*No (defiance)*	**No**/*No*
Moral acceptance of death—culture	**Yes**/*No*	**Yes**/*No*
	Spain/*USA*	**Spain**/*USA*

The philosophical underpinning of this construct is the perception that Western society is slowly coming to believe that a 'good death' implies cognitive acceptance of that same death, and this notion in itself is debatable. Also the perception that 'autonomy' of the patient always implies a cognitive acceptance of the impending death is debatable.

The differences in this table are overemphasized for the sake of clarity.

With no changes, this table has been published as in Núñez Olarte JM, Gracia Guillén D (2001). Cultural issues and ethical dilemmas in palliative and end-of-life care in Spain. *Cancer Control*, **8**, 46–54. The publisher's permission to reproduce the table has been gratefully acknowledged. Reproduced by permission from *Cancer Control: Journal of the Moffitt Cancer Centre.*

- Avoid generalization or stereotyping according to ethnic or cultural background.

- Be open to different approaches from minority groups within your culture, or from patients coming from other cultures.

- Consider information regarding your own and other cultures as essential for the well-being and optimal care of your patients.

- Be aware of the role, and potential influence, of the translator when needed.

- Promote changes in your organization: the word 'hospice' might be a barrier in itself.

- Recruit staff from minorities in order to reach and understand their culture.

Conclusion

There is always a danger of oversimplification when discussing cultural issues. An unbiased, honest, unprejudiced and an as-scientific-as-realistically-possible approach to them is essential. Cultural diversity is not a threatening phenomenon. It is certainly a challenge, because it introduces another level of complexity into our caring efforts, but simultaneously it exposes us to the full richness of the suffering human being.

References

Azoulay D, Brajtman S, Yehezkel M, Shahal-Gassner R, Cohen A (2000). When the family demands the discontinuation of morphine. *European Journal of Palliative Care*, 7, 138–40.

Bainbridge W and Baines E (2001). Insight into palliative care: an audience with the Dalai Lama. *European Journal of Palliative Care*, 8, 66–9.

Bates MS, Edwards WT, Anderson KO (1993). Ethnocultural influences on variation in chronic pain perception. *Pain*, 52, 101–12.

Bayés R, Limonero JT, Romero E, Arranz P (2000). *Medicina Clínica (Barc)*, 115, 579–82.

Berger JT, Rosner F, Potash J, Kark P, Benett AJ (2000). Communication in caring for terminally ill patients. *Journal of Palliative Medicine*, 3, 69–73.

Blackhall LJ, Murphy ST, Frank G, Michel V, Azen S (1995). Ethnicity and attitudes towards patient autonomy. *JAMA*, 274, 820–5.

Bruera E, Benisch-Tolley S, Hanson J, Calder K, Pituskin E (2000*a*). Patient's preferences versus physician perceptions of communication styles in palliative care. Abstract 12th MASCC International Symposium, 23–25 March 2000, Washington. *Supportive Care in Cancer*, 8, 258.

Bruera E, Neumann C, Mazzocato C, Sala R, Stiefel F (2000*b*). Attitudes and believes of palliative care physicians regarding communication with terminally ill cancer patients. *Palliative Medicine*, 14, 287–98.

Burn G (2001). A personal initiative to improve palliative care in India: 10 years on. *Palliative Medicine*, 15, 159–62.

Cabrera Bermudes C, Arenas López O, Bonilla Ibern M *et al.* (2000). Perfil del cuidador principal del enfermo atendido por equipos de Cuidados Paliativos: estudio multicéntrico descriptivo transversal. *Medicina Paliativa*, 7, 140–4.

Centeno Cortés C and Núñez Olarte JM (1994). Questioning diagnosis disclosure in terminal cancer patients: a prospective study evaluating patient's responses. *Palliative Medicine*, 8, 39–44.

Centeno Cortés C and Núñez Olarte JM (1998). Estudios sobre la comunicación del diagnóstico de cáncer en España. *Medicina Clínica (Barc)*, 110, 744–50.

Chan A and Woodruff R (1992). Palliative Care in a multicultural society: a comparison of the palliative care needs of English-speaking and non-English speaking patients. *Journal of Palliative Care*, 8, 69.

Charlton R, Dovey S, Mizushima Y, Ford E (1995). Attitudes to death and dying in the UK, New Zealand and Japan. *Journal of Palliative Care*, 11, 42–7.

Clark D (2001). European palliative care in the longue durée (editorial). *European Journal of Palliative Care*, 8, 92.

Clark D, ten Have H, Janssens R (2000). Common threads? Palliative care service developments in seven European countries. *Palliative Medicine*, 14, 479–90.

Cleeland CS, Gonin R, Baez L, Loehrer P, Pandya KJ (1997). Pain and treatment of pain in minority patients with cancer. *Annals of Internal Medicine*, 127, 813–16.

Couceiro A and Núñez Olarte JM (2001). Orientaciones para la sedación del enfermo terminal. *Medicina Paliativa*, 8, 138–43.

Curtis RJ, Patrick DL, Caldwell ES, Collier AC (2000). Why don't patients and physicians talk about end-of-life care. *Archives of Internal Medicine*, 160, 1690–6.

Dekkers W, Sandman L, Web P (2002). Good death or good life as a goal of palliative care. In H ten Have, D Clark, ed. *The Ethics of Palliative Care; European Perspectives*, pp. 106–125. Open University Press, Buckingham.

Edwards CL, Fillingim RB, Keefe F (2001). Race, ethnicity and pain. *Pain*, 94, 133–7.

Emanuel EJ, Fairclough DL, Emanuel LL (2000). Attitudes and desires related to euthanasia and physician-assisted suicide among terminally ill patient and their caregivers. *JAMA*, 284, 2460–8.

Fainsinger R, Waller A, Bercovici M *et al.* (2000). A multicentre international study of sedation for uncontrolled symptoms in terminally ill patients. *Palliative Medicine*, 14, 257–65.

Fetters MD and Masuda Y (2000). Japanese patients' preferences for receiving cancer test results while in the United States: introducing an advance directive for cancer disclosure. *Journal of Palliative Medicine*, 3, 361–74.

Field D and Copp G (1999). Communication and awareness about dying in the 1990s. *Palliative Medicine*, 13, 459–68.

Fielding R, Wong L, Ko L (1998). Strategies of information disclosure to Chinese cancer patients in an Asian community. *Psycho-oncology*, 7, 240–51.

Fonnegra de Jaramillo I (1992). Asistencia psicológica al paciente terminal. In PF Bejarano, I Jaramillo, ed. *Morir Con Dignidad*, pp. 221–42. Fundación Omega, Santa Fé de Bogotá.

Friedrichsen MJ, Strang PM, Carlsson ME (2000). Breaking bad news in the transition from curative to palliative cancer care—patients' view of the doctor giving the information. *Supportive Care in Cancer*, 8, 472–8.

Gonçalves JF and Castro S (2001). Diagnosis disclosure in a Portuguese oncological centre. *Palliative Medicine*, 15, 35–41.

Grassi L, Magnani K, Ercolani M (1999). Attitudes toward euthanasia and physician-assisted suicide among Italian primary care physicians. *Journal of Pain and Symptom Management*, 17, 188–96.

Grassi L, Giraldi T, Messina EG, Magnani K, Valle E, Cartei G (2000). Physicians' attitudes to and problems with truth-telling to cancer patients. *Supportive Care in Cancer*, 8, 40–5.

Hammes J (2000). The lessons from *Respecting your choices*. In MZ Solomon, AL Romer, KS Heller, ed. *Innovations in End-of-Life Care; Practical Strategies and International Perspectives*, pp.19–38. Mary Ann Liebert, Larchmont, New York.

Hosking M, Whiting G, Brathwate C, Fox P, Boshoff A, Robbins L (2000). Cultural attitudes towards death and dying: a South African perspective. *Palliative Medicine*, 14, 437–9.

Janssens R, ten Have H, Clark *et al.* (2001). Palliative care in Europe: towards a more comprehensive understanding. *European Journal of Palliative Care*, 8, 20–3.

Karim K, Bailey M, Tunna K (2000). Non-white ethnicity and the provision of specialist palliative care services: factors affecting doctors' referral patterns. *Palliative Medicine*, 14, 471–8.

Koffman J, Higginson IJ, Dunlop R (1999). Care in the last year of life: satisfaction with health services among the black Caribbean population in an inner London health authority. Research Abstract. *Palliative Medicine*, 13, 522–3.

Latimer EJ (2000). Cultural dimensions. In R Fisher, ed. *A Guide to End-of-Life Care for Seniors*. Sunnybrook Health Sciences Center, Toronto.

Lin CC (1999). Disclosure of the cancer diagnosis as it relates to the quality of pain management among patients with cancer pain in Taiwan. *Journal of Pain and Symptom Management*, 18, 331–7.

Lynn J (2000). Finding the key to reform in end-of-life care. *Journal of Pain and Symptom Management*, 19, 165–7.

Maddocks I. (2000) Teaching palliative care in East Asia. *Palliative Medicine*, 14, 535–7.

Mebane EW, Oman RF, Kroonen LT, Goldstein MK (1999). The influence of physician race, age and gender on physician attitudes toward advance care directives and preferences for end-of-life decision-making. *Journal of the American Geriatrics Society*, 47, 579–91.

Meseguer C, Luque JM, Conti M *et al.* (1995). Opiniones de los familiares sobre los cuidados paliativos recibidos. Estudio transversal de una muestra aleatoria simple de 154 familiares. Abstract en el I Congreso de la SECPAL. Barcelona, Spain. December 6–9, 1995. *Medicina Paliativa*, 2, 199.

Morita T (1999). Do hospice clinicians sedate patients intending to hasten death? *Journal of Palliative Care*, 15, 20–3.

Mystakidou K, Liossi C, Vlachos L, Papadimitriou J (1996). Disclosure of diagnostic information to cancer patients in Greece. *Palliative Medicine*, 10, 195–200.

Neuberger J (1998). Introduction. Cultural issues in palliative care. In D Doyle, G Hanks, and N MacDonald, eds. *Oxford Textbook of Palliative Medicine*. Second edition, pp. 777–85. Oxford University Press, Oxford.

Ngelangel CA *et al.* (1996). The process of disclosure in Philippine oncological practice. In *Thirteenth Asia Pacific Cancer Conference, Penang (Malaysia)*, p. 16. Abstract book. Practical Printers, Penang.

Núñez Olarte JM (1999). Care of the dying in 18th century Spain—the non-hospice tradition. *European Journal of Palliative Care*, 6, 23–7.

Núñez Olarte JM and Gracia Guillén D (2001). Cultural issues and ethical dilemmas in palliative and end-of-life care in Spain. *Cancer Control*, 8, 1–9.

Núñez Olarte JM and Fainsinger RL, de Moissac D (2000). Influencia de factores culturales en la estrategia de tratamiento. *Medicina Paliativa*, 7, 76–7.

Oliviere D (1999). Culture and ethnicity. *European Journal of Palliative Care*, 6, 53–6.

Pascual A and Gisbert A (2000). Sedación en una unidad de cuidados paliativos. Comunicación oral, III Congreso SECPAL, mayo 2000, Valencia. *Medicina Paliativa*, 7 (suppl. 1), 16.

Peruselli C, DiGiulio P, Toscani F *et al.* (1999). Home palliative care for terminal cancer patients: a survey on the final week of life. *Palliative Medicine*, 13, 233–41.

Pimentel FL, Maia-Goncalves JP, Mesquita NF, Vila-Real M, Silva-Ferreira J (2000). Truth telling to cancer patients in Portugal. Abstract 12th MASCC International Symposium, 23–25 March 2000, Washington. *Supportive Care in Cancer*, 8, 258.

Porta J, Guinovart C, Yllá-Catalá E *et al.* (1999). Definición y opiniones acerca de la sedación terminal: estudio multicéntrico catalano-balear. *Medicina Paliativa*, 6, 108–15.

Porta Sales J, Yllá-Catalá Boré E, Estíbalez Gil A *et al.* (1999). Estudio multicéntrico catalano-balear sobre la sedación terminal en Cuidados Paliativos. *Medicina Paliativa*, 6, 153–8.

Puchalski CM, Zhong Z, Jacobs MM *et al.* (2000). Patients who want their family and physician to make resuscitation decisions for them: observations from SUPPORT and HELP. *Journal of the American Geriatrics Society*, 48, S84–90.

Rebagliato M, Cuttini M, Broggin L *et al.* (2000). Neonatal end-of-life decision making. Physicians' attitudes and relationship with self-reported practices in 10 European countries. *JAMA*, 284, 2451–9.

Rosenfeld B, Breitbart W, Galietta M *et al.* (2000). The schedule of attitudes towards hastened death: measuring desire for death in terminally ill cancer patients. *Cancer*, 88, 2868–75.

Roy DJ (2000). Who really knows how to die? (editorial). *Journal of Palliative Care*, 16, 3–4.

Sapir R, Catane R, Kaufman B *et al.* (2000). Cancer patient expectations of and communication with oncologists and oncology nurses: the experience of an integrated oncology and palliative care service. *Supportive Care in Cancer*, 8, 458–63.

Seo M, Tamura K, Shijo H, Morioka E, Ikegame C, Hirasako K (2000). Telling the diagnosis to cancer patients in Japan: attitude of patients, physicians and nurses. *Palliative Medicine*, 14, 105–10.

Singer P, Martin D, Merrijoy K (1999). Quality end-of-life care. *JAMA*, **281**, 163–8.

Solomon MZ (2000). Why are advance directives a non-issue outside the United States? In MZ Solomon, AL Romer, KS Heller, ed. *Innovations in End-of-Life Care; Practical Strategies and International Perspectives*, pp. 13–18. Mary Ann Liebert, Larchmont, New York.

Spruyt O (1999). Community-based palliative care for Bangladeshi patients in east London. Accounts of bereaved carers. *Palliative Medicine*, **13**, 119–29.

Steinhauser KE, Christakis NA, Clipp EC, McNeilly M, McIntyre L, Tulsky JA (2000). Factors considered important at the end of life by patients, family, physicians, and other care providers. *JAMA*, **284**, 2476–82.

Steinhauser KE, Christakis NA, Clipp EC *et al.* (2001). Preparing for the end of life: preferences of patients, families, physicians, and other care providers. *Journal of Pain and Symptom Management*, **22**, 727–37.

Stone P, Phillips C, Spruyt O, Waight C (1997). A comparison of the use of sedatives in a hospital support team and in a hospice. *Palliative Medicine*, **11**, 140–4.

Tamburini M, Buccheri G, Brunelli C, Ferrigno D (2000). The difficult choice of chemotherapy in patients with unresectable non-small-cell lung cancer. *Supportive Care in Cancer*, **8**, 223–8.

Tylor EB (1971). *Primitive Culture*. John Murray, London.

Valera JP and Aubry R (2000). Morphine—doctors' beliefs and the myths. *European Journal of Palliative Care*, **7**, 178–82.

Viguria Arrieta JM, Rocafort Gil J, Eslava Gurrea E, Ortega Sobera M (2000). Sedación con midazolám. Eficacia de un protocolo de tratamiento en pacientes terminales con síntomas no controlables con otros medios. *Medicina Paliativa*, **7**, 2–5.

Yedidia MJ and MacGregor B (2001). Confronting the prospect of dying: reports of terminally ill patients. *Journal of Pain and Symptom Management*, **22**, 807–19.

7

Bereavement care

Marilyn Relf

Introduction

Supporting family members after bereavement is an integral part of palliative care and the majority of specialist services offer bereavement care. Individual support from volunteers is the usual strategy but written information, social and therapeutic groups, memorial services and counselling may also be available (Wilkes 1993). Although the need for bereavement services is widely recognized there is less consensus about the nature of services and how they should be delivered. There has been little systematic research and no agreement about the essential constituents of good practice.

Historically, the needs of bereaved people have been consistently underestimated with dedicated services set up only after nurses and other staff in palliative care settings have struggled to meet requests for on-going contact. It is tempting to conclude that, as services have been demand led, they will reflect the needs of users. To what extent is this true? This chapter will explore the factors that influence the ways in which we hear and respond to the voices of bereaved people.

Fundamental to the delivery of bereavement care, whatever strategies of support are adopted, is the ability to listen accurately to what people say about their experiences. Although listening is part of everyday life, it is not a neutral activity. In practice we filter what people say through lenses provided by our knowledge, training and personal experiences. What we 'hear' is a result of this process. Theories and models provide us with conceptual maps of 'normal' and 'complicated' grief and social constructs influence our perceptions of need. For example, it may be assumed that members of minority groups will always have support from their 'community' with the result that individual needs may remain unexplored. Similarly, bereaved people 'hear' us through their lenses such as notions of 'good grief' or 'manly' behaviour. Hearing the voices of bereaved people is a complex process.

Theories and models of grief

Theories and models provide conceptual frameworks that help us to make sense of what we hear. The rationale for involving volunteers draws on stress theory and the role of social support as a mediator between stress and health deterioration (Payne *et al.* 1999). Bereavement has serious health consequences for a substantial minority of people (Stroebe and Stroebe 1987) and deprives individuals of the direct support provided by the deceased. Joint suffering and differential expressions of grief within a social network may also reduce the amount of support available. A perceived lack of social support is a major risk factor associated with poor adaptation to bereavement (Stylianos and Vachon 1993). Intervention, therefore, is conceptualized as compensating for deficits in informal support in order to prevent or ameliorate health risks.

Studies of the relationship between social support and health conclude that emotional support and information are the factors that make a difference. These promote self-esteem, provide reassurance and enable people to think through their problems (Cohen and Wills 1985). Supportive listening rather than therapeutic counselling, therefore, is likely to be sufficient to help the majority of people cope with bereavement. Indeed, all 'bereavement counselling' should be non-intrusive and rooted in the ' ... basic and spontaneous comfort of one human being for another' (Raphael 1980). Parkes (1980) in a review of studies of the effectiveness of bereavement counselling endorses this view and concludes that volunteers may rival professionals in their ability to provide proactive bereavement care. Volunteer support may also be more acceptable as it lacks the stigma associated with mental health provision and indicates that grief is not an illness.

According to stress theory, support will only be needed if the demands of a situation exceed the available resources. On-going support is unlikely, therefore, to be needed by all bereaved people. In order to assess vulnerability and target services, Parkes designed a risk index utilizing research on the risk factors associated with poor health following bereavement (see Parkes and Weiss 1983). Risk assessment is widely used in palliative care (Payne and Relf 1994) and this practice will be discussed further later in this chapter. The rationale for palliative care bereavement services, therefore, is continuity of support to vulnerable people as a preventive health care measure by providing emotional support and information about grief.

What evidence is there that the methods adopted meet the needs of users? Unfortunately studies of the effectiveness of bereavement services focus on comparing the health of supported and unsupported people. The interventions provided have been neglected and we have little understanding of how bereaved people use support or what makes a difference.

The work of bereavement services is often described as 'bereavement counselling', users referred to as 'clients' and both voluntary and paid workers referred to as 'counsellors'. I have discussed the use of the term 'counselling' for proactive support elsewhere (Payne *et al.* 1999). Although the training of volunteers usually includes counselling skills it rarely meets the accreditation criteria for counsellors required by organizations such as the British Association of Counselling. In this chapter, I use 'support' to distinguish supportive counselling from therapeutic counselling, 'users' rather than 'clients' and 'helpers' to refer to those providing support.

Models of grief derived from psychoanalytic and attachment theories and from empirical studies of widows have had a major influence on the delivery of bereavement care (see Payne *et al.* 1999). To summarize, successful adaptation is conceptualized as relating to the degree to which mourners complete a process of adjustment consisting of overlapping phases, stages or tasks. A central notion is that grief must be expressed otherwise it will be manifested in some other way, often depression (Bowlby 1981). Many bereaved people, and their helpers, believe that it is a fact that grief proceeds in stages and descriptions of bereavement counselling stress the necessity of enabling people to express their feelings and to work through their grief to avoid a pathological outcome (Lendrum and Syme 1992; Faulkner 1995). According to Wortman and Silver (1989) normality is defined by this view; this is the 'clinical lore' of bereavement support. Worden (1983), for example, stresses the need to encourage bereaved people to complete four tasks: accept the reality of the death, experience emotional pain, adjust to all the changes caused by the loss and detach emotional energy from the deceased in order to move on with life. Although his third task includes learning new roles and skills, the emphasis is on the psychological dimension. In short, according to this view grief is similar to an illness; offering support proactively may prevent the wound becoming infected while reactive intervention aims to provide a 'cure'.

How useful is the grief work model for proactive services? An evaluation of a palliative care service found that this model was helpful but not sufficient as a framework for intervention. Relf (1997, 2000) undertook a randomized, controlled study comparing the health outcomes of supported and unsupported 'at-risk' bereaved people and also explored the experiences of receiving and providing support from the perspectives of both bereaved people and volunteers. The results confirmed Parkes' conclusion (Parkes 1981) that targeted proactive volunteer support is effective. People in the intervention group were less anxious and were significantly less likely to increase their use of health care, particularly general practitioners. This method of evaluation, however, assumes that intervention is similar to a drug with the 'dose' being the same for all. The qualitative findings revealed that reactions to support varied. Three-quarters of the intervention group welcomed support and used it extensively. Four themes describe what they experienced as helpful: being able to talk about their loss, feeling understood, talking to someone who was outside their social network and information about grief. They talked openly about the events leading up to the death, reminisced about their life with the deceased, explored their emotional responses, sought reassurance that their reactions were 'normal' and discussed how to manage all the changes triggered by bereavement. The volunteers described supporting such people as relatively easy despite the depth of emotion or complexity of problems. There was a good match between their expectations of their role and the needs of the people they were visiting.

A quarter of those who had received support were less sure that it had been helpful. They had less contact with the service, were not so overtly distressed and described support in social terms; what they valued was 'general chat' although some stated that this had neglected their 'real' problems. A minority expressed dissatisfaction; they experienced support as a painful reminder of all they were attempting to keep under control. The volunteers found it more difficult to develop rapport with these groups. They did not want to be intrusive or to press them to confront their feelings as suggested by phase models of grief. They wondered how much 'grief work' is necessary and whether not exploring feelings was a way of coping that could be helpful rather than problematic. In particular they did not want to undermine ways of coping that were not perceived as problematic by users.

Phase models describe the major themes of grief and were not intended to be used as prescriptive models of intervention. The experiences of younger widows had a strong influence on early models of grief and more recent research, including other groups of bereaved people, has prompted critical re-appraisal and theoretical development. The accumulating evidence is that people vary in the way they perceive, experience, express and cope with bereavement. Advances in understanding that enable us to understand users' responses to bereavement services include the following.

Continuing bonds

The concept that adjustment depends on severing attachment to the deceased in order to 'move on' has been misconstrued as a process of forgetting rather than a process of changing the nature of the attachment. Studies of childhood and parental grief show that bereaved people do not see themselves as relinquishing attachment bonds but describe a process of negotiating and re-negotiating the meaning of the lost relationship over time, constructing new connections to the deceased (Klass *et al.* 1996). Important relationships continue to influence present reality whether the person is physically present or not. This means that there may not be a definite end point that marks 'recovery' or 'closure'.

Walter (1996) argues that the traditional emphasis on the emotional dimension of grief may result in bereaved people being discouraged from talking about the deceased and thus denied the opportunity to discover and integrate the meaning of the relationship. His biographical model of grief emphasizes the importance of talking to others about the deceased.

Coping

The Dual Process Model of Grief (Stroebe and Schut 1999) proposes that bereaved people oscillate between feelings of loss and managing life without the deceased. Loss orientation encompasses the emotional expressions of grief described in traditional models: sorrow, pining, thinking about the deceased and holding on to memories. Restoration orientation encompasses regulating emotions in order to master the tasks and roles performed by the deceased, make lifestyle adjustments and build a new identity. Personality factors, gender and cultural background will influence the dominant mode and the degree to which each individual oscillates. At first behaviour is likely to be more loss focused but over time the balance shifts towards restoration. This model enables helpers to understand that emotional control is functional and that it is important to listen to, and support, restoration orientation as well as loss orientation.

Martin and Doka (2000) describe the importance of personality in determining the experience and expression of grief. They view grief as a continuum with two dominant patterns. People who are primarily in touch with their feelings experience 'intuitive grief', waves of intense feelings as described in the traditional models. People who are primarily in touch with their thoughts, however, experience grief as a cognitive process or 'instrumental grief'. For example, instrumental mourners cope by seeking information, thinking through problems, taking action and seeking diversion.

Martin and Doka suggest that bereavement services are more likely to meet the needs of intuitive mourners and that instrumental mourners may be viewed as deviant and disenfranchised. They argue that neither pattern of grief is superior and that helpers should enable people to build on their strengths while helping them to develop their range of coping strategies. Helpers may act as confidants but they also act as 'sounding boards' enabling thoughts to be clarified and problems addressed.

Social norms

Although grief is universal, the way it is experienced and expressed varies across cultures (Parkes *et al.* 1997). For example, people in late modern societies such as the UK may be socialized to value self-reliance, independence and autonomy more than revealing vulnerability and weakness. In particular men experience pressure to suppress emotions and hide distress. However, although grief may be influenced by gender, it is not determined by it (Martin and Doka 2000). For example, Riches and Dawson (1997) report that, following the death of a child, the conventional distinctions between men and women could not account for the range of behaviours they observed. Some fathers expressed their emotions freely whereas some mothers exhibited 'male' coping styles. Eichenbaum and Orbach (1983) also report that many women feel ashamed for needing support and may equate this with weakness and childishness. Helpers should be wary of making assumptions based on gender and recognize that personality and coping strategies may be more important.

Walter (1999) describes the prevailing norms that regulate mourning in late modern societies as focusing on emotional control; grief should be conducted in private and only hinted at in public. He argues that the belief that healthy grief is emotionally expressive exists in tension with these norms. Indeed, Walter suggests that bereavement supporters may become 'grief police' imposing expressive behaviour. Walter's description of private mourning may explain why some people may be reluctant to accept support. People may present themselves in line with societal expectations and there may be a discrepancy between public expressions and on-going distress (Tait and Silver 1989). Helpers, therefore, need to be highly skilled at forming relationships.

Adopting a multi-dimensional framework of intervention may be useful (see Parkes *et al.* 1996). This approach conceptualizes grief as having social, physical, spiritual, practical and behavioural dimensions as well being a psychological process. It recognizes that people have strengths to help them cope and enables helpers to perceive their role as understanding and empowering bereaved people rather than monitoring progress. It enables helpers to 'hear' how 'this loss' is affecting 'this person'. Case study 1 illustrates many of the emerging themes in our understanding of grief. Jack did not choose to focus on his emotional reactions but was immersed in finding the meaning of his relationship with his wife. His grief may be described as predominantly instrumental and his focus changed from the past to his future after he had constructed a 'true' account of his relationship with his wife. The case study also illustrates the role of supervision in enabling Jack's volunteer to recognize her own feelings of difference and to understand his needs.

Case study 1

Jack's wife, Charlotte, died after a short illness. He saw Ellen, a bereavement service volunteer, nine times. He focused on his relationship with his wife, showing Ellen videotapes, photos and letters. He also reported back on his discussions about Charlotte with friends, how they had perceived her and what she had meant to them. After the third visit Ellen told her supervisor that she had decided to close; Jack was able to talk to others, was not emotional and did not need her help. In discussion it emerged that Jack made Ellen feel redundant. He was articulate, talked non-stop and did not seem to hear what she said. He moved in a very different social circle, his friends were 'important' people including a psychoanalyst and a psychiatrist and he was an able and successful man. Consequently Ellen felt anxious and clumsy in her responses. The supervisor suggested discussing her role with Jack. To Ellen's surprise, he was very keen for her visits to continue. Her support enabled him to piece things together in his mind and, as she had never met Charlotte, he could be totally frank. At the next meeting Jack talked about his discovery of Charlotte's love affairs, the hurts that he had endured and his self-doubts. Perhaps he had never been as important to her as she was to him. This thought was unbearable. This conversation changed the relationship. Both Jack and Ellen became more relaxed and began to 'hear' each other. When Ellen did close it was with a sense of genuine affection and delight that Jack's attention had turned to the present and on building a new life.

Communication skills

Variations in coping styles may influence the use of support but the ability of helpers to work *with* rather than *on* bereaved people also depends on the quality of their communication skills. Although the focused use of everyday interpersonal skills is at the centre of all 'helping relationships', helpful relationships go beyond ordinary discourse (Egan 1994; Hawkins and Shohet 2000). Of fundamental importance is the ability to demonstrate openness, respect and non-judgemental acceptance combined with warmth and empathy (Rogers 1961). Adopting these core values enables attention to be given to the individual nature of each person's grief and reduces the likelihood of service users feeling that they have not been 'heard'. Listening in this way means that assumptions will be constantly revised through experience and that respect for diversity will become central to service provision. Parkes et al. (1996) describe the use of communication skills to demonstrate these values and enable helpers to build relationships. However, a number of factors may prevent helpers from doing so.

Coping

As described earlier coping styles vary. Some bereaved people will prefer to be independent or seek to maintain emotional control.

Attitudes of helpers

Helpers' attitudes are also shaped by their personality and past experiences. What has been their experience of grief? Are they more at home with their feelings or their thoughts? How might their attitudes influence their expectations of others? Training programmes should raise awareness that assumptions about others may be influenced by factors such as age, gender, class and ethnicity.

Experience

Experience makes a difference (Parkes 1981). Relf (2000) found that inexperienced volunteers were more anxious, worrying that they might cause further distress, whereas experienced volunteers were more open and empathic. Anxiety reduces the ability to listen and respond and seems to be widespread in interactions with bereaved people (Lehman et al. 1986). Even newly qualified professional counsellors demonstrate low levels of empathy when encountering grief (Kirchberg et al. 1998). Bereavement services should anticipate helpers' anxiety and address this in training and supervision.

Lack of information

Bereaved people may be anxious about accepting support. This may reflect sensitivity to rejection or fear of being pressed into intimacy (Kalish 1985). Not knowing what to expect is unhelpful (Pierce 1996) and people need information in order to understand what is being offered. Volunteers may find it difficult to explain their role (Relf 2000; Rowley and Littleford 1995) and there is a danger that users may form inaccurate assumptions. For example, there are similarities between the early stages of helping relationships and friendship. If users think that friendship is being offered, the eventual withdrawal of support may cause further loss (Faulkner 1995). Bereavement services should provide leaflets describing the service, the training and supervision of helpers, the code of confidentiality, what and how records are kept and the complaints procedure. Bereaved people need to have control over intervention (Stroebe and Stroebe 1987). One way of achieving this is to suggest four or five meetings and then review the utility of support (Parkes *et al.* 1996).

Need for professional counselling

Supportive listening will not always be appropriate. There may be complex problems that predate bereavement. It is important that services do not require volunteers to work beyond their competence. Services should have access to different levels of expertise both for guidance and to enable appropriate referrals to be made.

Impact of the work

The complexity of reactions and the deep sense of inner disturbance can be frightening for both bereaved people and those attempting to provide support. Supporters often feel helpless; it is impossible to bring back the deceased (Parkes 1986) and the work may confront them with situations that they dread (Raphael 1980). For example, this may include listening to detailed descriptions of disfiguring disease or mutilating surgery. The work provides a stark reminder that we are likely to lose those we love. There is also a risk of over-involvement or of personal grief being reawakened (Raphael *et al.* 1993). As case study 1 illustrated, helpers need to be able to recognize when their ability to respond is becoming blocked by their own reactions.

Self-awareness

Being able to respond helpfully to others relies on developing a high degree of self-awareness. It is important that all those who choose to work with bereaved people reflect on their motivations. Neglecting to do so increases the danger of dabbling in people's lives in order to meet our own needs. Two areas demand exploration. Firstly, to what extent does working in an area that is often viewed as 'special' fulfil a desire to be seen as a 'good person' in the eyes of others? Secondly, what idealistic projections does the worker hold about the role they hope to fulfil? Little is known about the motivation of bereavement service volunteers but it is likely that personal experience is important. People frequently choose to volunteer in settings connected to their personal lives (Lynn and Davis Smith 1991) and experience of bereavement is an important motivator for general hospice volunteers (Field and Johnson 1993). It is important to enable helpers to explore the interface between their personal reactions and assumptions and the work. This is facilitated by training and particularly by supervision.

Supervision

People who are involved in helping relationships usually respond positively to support and encouragement and want to develop their competence and monitor their practice. If this is ignored, practice will become unsafe for both bereaved people and their helpers. Supervision has three functions: support, education and management. It provides the infrastructure to enable individuals to discuss the impact of their work, enhance their competence and work within agreed limits (Hawkins and Shohet 2000).

Support

Helpers may fear that they are not good enough, they may become personally distressed by the work or overwhelmed by feelings of helplessness. Support enables them to carry on being open to others by providing regular opportunities to share the responsibility, off-load anxieties, explore personal reactions, regain perspective and feel reassured and empowered to carry on. Without support, helpers may either carry on absorbing distress until they become overwhelmed or protect themselves by distancing from the work. A lack of support increases the risk that helpers burn out.

Education

This aspect of supervision enables helpers to carry on learning and developing. It enables them to conceptualize in new ways, to clarify their intentions, to consider the interventions they are using and to explore other options. Without this aspect of supervision, helpers may become stale.

Management

This ensures safety, accountability, that standards are put into practice, that the work is ethical and that resources are used appropriately. Standards and ethical principles for bereavement services have recently been outlined by

Hartley (2001) and it is important that supervisors enable helpers to work within agreed limits. This aspect of supervision includes ensuring that helpers recognize the need to take time off when facing stressful events in their own lives. It also encompasses organizational issues such as involving helpers in decision-making processes.

Service co-ordination

As the previous discussion indicates, co-ordination is an important aspect of service provision. It encompasses service planning and evaluation, managing referrals, recruiting and selecting voluntary and paid staff and ensuring that training and supervision are provided. Risk assessment plays a central part in ensuring that the differing needs of bereaved people are recognized.

Assessment of need

In pro-active services, risk assessment is concerned with targeting support to meet diverse needs. The practice recognizes that many people will have sufficient support from their social networks and aims to ensure that resource allocation is consistent and objective. Many services use assessment tools derived from Parkes' risk index (see Parkes and Weiss 1983) and based on risk factors associated with poor health following bereavement (Payne and Relf 1994). There are three groups of risk factors: the circumstances surrounding the death, the personality of the bereaved person and the availability of social support (see Parkes *et al.* 1996). Using formal methods ensures that needs are assessed routinely but there are a number of problems with assessment tools. Firstly, the evidence that Parkes' risk index is a reliable and valid predictive tool is limited (Beckwith *et al.* 1990; Levy *et al.* 1992). Secondly, there may be little time for nurses to get to know families sufficiently well to be able to assess need and family needs may be given low priority (Field *et al.* 1992). Lastly, the focus is on indicators of pathology and indicators of resilience are neglected (Payne and Relf 1994). These limitations mean that assessment tools should not be used alone but as part of a process involving training assessors, making assessment a team responsibility and drawing on the clinical experience of service co-ordinators. As well as reaching out to those who may be at risk, it is also important to ensure that services are accessible to all bereaved people. It is good practice to provide clear, jargon-free written information to facilitate self-referral. It is important that service providers continue the process of assessment to ensure that support is appropriate to users' needs.

Helpers should know what other services are available and how to enable users to access them.

Case study 2

Colin died at home after a short illness. Risk assessment identified that his wife, Joan, should be offered support as she was now the sole carer for Mary, their severely disabled adult daughter. After several sessions it became clear that Mary was eager to have support herself. She saw her volunteer 11 times. They met at Mary's day centre where the staff ensured that they had a room to themselves. Mary communicated through an electronic memo pad, displaying only five words at a time. Communication was slow but Mary talked about her father, his illness, the funeral, how much he meant to her, her pride in his achievements and her anger that he was no longer with her. She expressed her sadness, her worries about her mother and her fears for her future. The volunteer described how she used her skills to overcome the distance the typing created. She found it important to sit in a position where she could both read what was being written and also be seen by Mary. She realized that she must not make assumptions about what Mary was typing but wait until she had finished. She needed to regularly check out the accuracy of her understanding. Silences were hard to interpret; sometimes Mary stopped because she was in physical pain. Her eyes became sore and it was hard to tell when she was crying. The decision to end was mutual; Mary continued to be sad at times and to worry about her future but felt much more at ease with her loss and was enjoying many aspects of her life. The volunteer often talked about Mary in her monthly supervision sessions. She felt strongly that Mary's needs might have been overlooked. Why was Mary not included in the risk assessment process? Was it assumed that because she looked different her grief would be different or that her communication problems would prevent her from using support? These questions prompted the staff to reflect on their decision making and raised awareness of the needs of people with disabilities.

Service evaluation

Audit and evaluation should be on-going in order to monitor, review and learn from the experience of service delivery. Evaluation should include all the stakeholders in service provision: bereaved people, volunteers and paid staff, supervisors, those with responsibility for risk assessment and palliative care managers. Whereas it is relatively easy to monitor service use, obtaining stakeholders' views may be more complex. However, this is an important aspect of ensuring that services are sensitive, user-responsive and cost-effective. A variety of methods may be used.

Research

Traditionally research has primarily focused on developing theories and evaluating interventions by measuring and comparing the health of supported and unsupported bereaved people. These quantitative methods have neglected users' views. Qualitative methods enable the 'real world' of service provision to be described and explored. Such methods are described elsewhere (see Clark 1997) and provide rich insights into service use. For example, Riches and Dawson (2000) used both participant observation and interviews to explore parental loss and Relf (2000) used semi-structured interviews to explore the work of volunteer support workers. Users may be involved in research in a number of ways. For example, they can be members of advisory groups to help identify and define areas for exploration and they can collaborate by giving regular feedback on work in progress and by contributing to the analysis and interpretation of findings. They can be included in the dissemination and discussion of findings by being invited to participate in conferences. Riches and Dawson (2000) collaborated with three groups of stakeholders by inviting bereaved parents, bereavement workers and researchers to seminars and presentations in order to obtain feedback on their emerging research findings. Silverman (1988) also describes this process of refining ideas through discourse with user groups as well as 'expert' clinicians and theorists. Such collaboration helps research to remain open to real experience and avoids experts misrepresenting users' voices (Riches and Dawson 2000). The findings gain greater credibility because they represent a coming together of different voices, insights and influences. The nature of bereavement means that there are particular ethical issues that need to be addressed when conducting research with bereaved people. Those involved in research need to understand how to respond to expressions of grief and be provided with supervision to enable them to avoid becoming over involved or too detached. Parkes (1995) discusses these difficulties and provides ethical guidelines for conducting bereavement research. Many services have little time or resources to undertake formal research. It may be possible, however, to build links with academic institutions and experienced researchers who can provide guidance and expertise. Organizations in the UK such as the Palliative Care Research Society and the Bereavement Research Forum provide opportunities to network with people who are grappling with the complexities of service evaluation.

Needs assessment

This enables assumptions about need to be checked out and gives users a voice in service planning. It involves identifying stakeholders, seeking their opinions about current practice and comparing these with recognized examples of good practice. Several methods can be used including interviews, surveys, focus groups and participant observation. For example, before setting up a service for bereaved children, a palliative care service interviewed bereaved young people, parents and professionals such as teachers, school nurses, educational psychologists and social workers. The findings confirmed that parents and young people experienced a lack of accessible information and support. It also revealed a need for advice and training among professionals. An advisory group of stakeholders was set up and a strategy to address the identified needs was adopted. The needs assessment made an important contribution to successful fund raising and provided a base line to audit the actual use of the new service against expressed needs. For example, at the first year review, activity figures showed that the service was receiving more requests for support than had been anticipated from families facing bereavement and a strategy was devised to respond to this need.

Involving users

This gives users a direct voice in service review and delivery. Forums enable services to consult with users, for example to obtain feedback on the clarity or relevance of written information or to obtain the opinions of particular groups such as teenagers or ethnic minority groups. Users may also directly participate in service provision, for example, by becoming trustees or members of management groups, by running mutual support groups or by becoming volunteers.

Obtaining feedback from users

A number of methods are available. Feedback forms may be used to gather information routinely (Pierce 1996). Forms may use rating scales or seek opinions, for example, about what was helpful or less helpful or what might be improved. Focus groups may be set up to enable users to discuss their experience of support. It is important to remember that satisfaction does not necessarily ensure quality and that focus groups provide a multiplicity of views rather than a 'typical' voice. The argument that views are not representative may be used to question the validity of user feedback and it may be difficult to balance the view that every individual voice is valid with the need to make decisions about the use of resources to meet collective needs. There is a danger that louder voices may dominate and priorities set accordingly. As illustrated in case study 2, some groups of users may have small voices but considerable needs. It is also important to seek feedback from people who choose not to become users and who refuse or make little use of services.

Involving others

Organizations need to involve helpers as well as users in planning and decision making. One advantage of volunteers is that they have often been bereaved themselves, they may be former users, they are members of the local community and they bring a wide range of experiences and views that enrich the work. Recruitment can target particular groups to create a team that reflects the diversity within the communities they serve. Involving volunteers also helps to ensure that professional perspectives do not dominate services.

In general consulting widely and in different ways is desirable so that resource allocation and practice reflects users' views as well as clinical lore and research evidence. Whatever methods of participation are adopted it is important to be sensitive to the circumstances of bereaved people who may be preoccupied with grief.

♦ Being consulted may be stressful, particularly if choices have to be made about the use of resources.

♦ Grief is influenced by social norms and bereaved people may express views that they believe to be socially desirable. For example, they may minimize their reactions because they believe that they should not dwell on grief.

♦ Users may be influenced by their experience of palliative care before bereavement. For example, they may feel obliged to participate and to give positive feedback because of the care given to the deceased.

♦ It is important to be sensitive to the grief process; bereavement is associated with strong emotions and impaired thinking processes. Attending groups may be stressful, particularly in the early months following bereavement. Views may change during the course of bereavement and reflect the timing of consultations.

Conclusion

This chapter has discussed a number of factors that influence the way that we hear and respond to the voices of bereaved people. It has been argued that listening to others is not a neutral activity and that what people say is filtered through lenses provided by conceptual frameworks, personal experiences of loss and the quality of communication skills. These lenses influence the way that bereaved people's voices are heard, whether we are offering support or seeking their participation in service planning, delivery or evaluation. Skilled listening remains central to understanding the meaning of what people tell us about their experiences and structures need to be in place to prepare and support all those involved in understanding bereavement. The experiences of bereaved people may be explored using qualitative research methods and findings have contributed to recent theoretical developments. These include recognizing the importance of continuing bonds, understanding the cognitive processes involved in grief, that avoidance is an effective coping strategy, and recognizing the influence of social norms on ways of coping. A number of other ways of involving users have been described in order to plan, evaluate and refine bereavement care. Support workers also have a role in such explorations. It is important that the voices of both helpers and users join those of expert clinicians, researchers and theorists. Including all those involved will help to develop flexible, responsive services sensitive to diversity in the experience and expression of grief.

References

Beckwith, B.E., Beckwith, S.K., Gray, T.L., Micsko, M.M., Holm, J.E., Plummer, V.H., Flaa, S.L. (1990). Identification of spouses at high risk during bereavement: a preliminary assessment of Parkes and Weiss' risk index. *The Hospice Journal* 6: 35–45.

Bowlby, J. (1981). *Attachment and Loss: Volume 3, Loss, Sadness and Depression.* Harmondsworth: Penguin.

Clark, D. (1997). What is qualitative research and what can it contribute to palliative care? *Palliative Medicine* 11: 159–66.

Cohen, S., Wills, T.A. (1985). Stress, social support and the buffering hypothesis. *Psychological Bulletin* 98: 310–57.

Eichenbaum, L., Orbach, S. (1983) *Understanding Women.* London: Penguin.

Egan, G. (1994). *The Skilled Helper: A Problem Management Approach to Helping.* Fifth edition. Pacific Grove, California: Brooks Cole.

Faulkner, A. (1995). *Working with Bereaved People.* Edinburgh: Churchill Livingstone.

Field, D., Johnson, I. (1993). Volunteers in the British hospice movement. In Clark, D. (ed.) *The Sociology of Death.* Oxford: Blackwell Publishers, pp. 198–217.

Field, D., Dand, P., Ahmedzai, S., Biswas, B. (1992). Care and information received by lay carers of terminally ill patients at the Leicestershire Hospice. *Palliative Medicine* 6: 237–45.

Hartley, J. (2001). *Standards for Bereavement Care in the UK*. London: London Bereavement Network.

Hawkins, P., Shohet, R. (2000). *Supervision in the Helping Professions*. Second edition. Buckingham: Open University Press.

Kalish, R.A. (1985). *Death, Grief and Caring Relationships*. Second edition. California: Brooks Cole.

Kirchberg, T.M., Niemayer, R.A., James, R.K. (1998). Beginning counsellors' death concerns and empathic responses to client situations involving death and grief. *Death Studies* 22: 99–120.

Klass, D., Silverman, P.R., Nickman, S.L. (1996). *Continuing Bonds*. Washington: Taylor and Francis.

Lehman, D.R., Ellard, J.H., Wortman, C.B. (1986). Social support for the bereaved: recipients' and providers' perspectives on what is helpful. *Journal of Consulting and Clinical Psychology* 54: 438–46.

Lendrum, S., Syme, G. (1992). *Gift of Tears*. London: Routledge.

Levy, L.H., Derby, J.F., Martinowski, K.S. (1992). The question of who participates in bereavement research and the bereavement risk index. *Omega—Journal of Death and Dying* 25: 225–38.

Lynn, P., Davis Smith, J. (1991). *The 1991 National Survey of Voluntary Activity in the UK*. Voluntary Action Research, Second Series, Paper 1. Berkhamsted: The Volunteer Centre, UK.

Martin, T.L., Doka, K.J. (2000). *Men Don't Cry … Women Do*. Philadelphia: Taylor and Francis.

Parkes, C.M. (1980). Bereavement counselling: does it work? *British Medical Journal* 281: 3–6.

Parkes, C.M. (1981). Evaluation of a bereavement service. *Journal of Preventive Psychiatry* 1: 179–88.

Parkes, C.M., Weiss, R.S. (1983). *Recovery From Bereavement*. New York: Basic Books.

Parkes, C.M. (1986). *Bereavement. Studies of grief in adult life*. 2nd edition. London: Penguin.

Parkes, C.M. (1995). Guidelines for conducting ethical bereavement research. *Death Studies* 19: 171–81.

Parkes, C.M., Relf, M., Couldrick, A. (1996). *Counselling in Terminal Care and Bereavement*. Leicester: BPS Books.

Parkes, C.M., Laungani, P., Young, B. (1997). *Death and Bereavement Across Cultures*. London: Routledge.

Payne, S., Relf, M. (1994). A survey of bereavement needs assessment and support services. *Palliative Medicine* 8: 291–7.

Payne, S., Horn, S., Relf, M. (1999). *Loss and Bereavement*. Buckingham: Open University Press.

Pierce, G. (1996). Developing a client feedback system. In Machin, L., Pierce, G. (ed.) *Research: A Route to Good Practice*. Keele: University of Keele, Centre for Counselling Studies, pp. 36–57.

Raphael, B. (1980). A psychiatric model for counselling. In Schoenberg, B.M. (ed.) *Bereavement Counselling a Multidisciplinary Handbook*. Connecticut: Greenwood Press, pp. 147–172.

Raphael, B., Middleton, W., Martinek, N., Misso, V. (1993). Counselling and therapy of the bereaved. In Stroebe, M.S., Stroebe, W., Hansson, R.O. (ed.) *Handbook of Bereavement*. Cambridge: Cambridge University Press, pp. 427–53.

Relf, M. (1997). How effective are volunteers in providing bereavement care? In De Conno, F. (ed.) *Proceedings of the Fourth Congress of the European Association for Palliative Care*. 6/9 December 1995, Barcelona. Milan: EAPC, pp. 244–9.

Relf, M. (2000). The effectiveness of volunteer bereavement care. An evaluation of a palliative care bereavement service. Unpublished PhD Thesis, University of London.

Riches, G., Dawson, P. (1997). Shoring up the walls of heartache: parental responses to the death of a child. In Field, D. Hockey, J., Small, N. (ed.) *Death, Gender and Ethnicity*. London: Routledge, pp. 52–75.

Riches, G., Dawson, P. (2000). *An Intimate Loneliness*. Buckingham: Open University Press.

Rogers, C.R. (1961). *On Becoming a Person*. London: Constable.

Rowley, J., Littleford, A. (1995). An overview of bereavement counselling. *Palliative Care Today* 4: 21–2.

Silverman, P. (1988). Research as process: exploring the meaning of widowhood. In Reinharz, S., Rowles, D. (ed.) *Qualitative Gerontology*. New York: Springer, pp. 217–40.

Stroebe, M.S., Schut, H. (1999). The dual process model of coping with bereavement: rationale and description. *Death Studies* 23: 197–224.

Stroebe, W., Stroebe, M.S. (1987). *Bereavement and Health*. Cambridge: Cambridge University Press.

Stylianos, S.K., Vachon, M.L.S. (1993). The role of social support in bereavement. In Stroebe, M.S., Stroebe, W., Hansson, R.O. (ed.) *Handbook of Bereavement: Theory, Research and Intervention*. Cambridge: Cambridge University Press, pp. 397–410.

Tait, R., Silver, R.C. (1989). Coming to terms with major negative life events. In Uleman, J.S., Bargh, J.A. (ed.) *Unintended Thought*. New York: Guilford Press, pp. 351–82.

Walter, T. (1996). A new model of grief: bereavement and biography. *Mortality* 1: 7–25.

Walter, T. (1999). *On Bereavement: The Culture of Grief.* Milton Keynes: Open University Press.

Wilkes, E. (1993). Characteristics of hospice bereavement services. *Journal of Cancer Care* 2: 183–9.

Worden, J.W. (1983). *Grief Counselling and Grief Therapy.* London: Tavistock.

Wortman, C.B., Silver, R.C. (1989). The myths of coping with loss. *Journal of Consulting and Clinical Psychology* 57: 349–57.

Part 2

Multi-professional perspectives

8

Multi-professional teamwork

Pam Firth

Introduction

The provision of specialist palliative care for dying patients needs to acknowledge that the patient is central in the unit of care and that generally family members provide most of the care and will therefore need help and support themselves. A single worker in this situation has an impossible task to meet these needs without the skills of other professionals.

Palliative care is normally delivered by multi-professional teams whose composition can vary but usually have core personnel such as doctors, nurses, social workers and chaplains. They can and frequently do utilize the skills of others when necessary.

In the UK a series of tragedies involving children and adults led to public enquiries that highlighted the need for better communication and co-ordination of services for children and vulnerable adults. Co-operation between health services, social services and education were highlighted as areas of concern and recognition of the need to work together was emphasized. There is recognition that people with multiple health and social needs require professionals to co-operate across professional and service boundaries.

Loxley (1997, cited in Payne 2000) identifies 25 different Acts and government documents between 1970 and 1990 and 10 national, professional co-ordinating bodies concerned in some way with co-operation between health and social services.

The chapter will start with a brief overview of the development of multi-professional working in hospitals and the community. It will go on to examine what is meant by teams and teamworking and will look at some of the reasons for conflict. It will consider the development of hospices, specialist palliative care teams and the way in which these operate as systems, and consider the challenges, dilemmas and opportunities for multi-professional teamwork.

What is meant by multi-professional teamwork?

Multi-professional, multi-disciplinary, inter-professional—what do we mean? Øvretveit *et al.* (1997) state that in 15 years they have worked with 134 groups, each of which called themselves a multi-disciplinary team, but there were differences in the way all of these teams worked and the authors discovered that making assumptions about working practices was not helpful. The danger in defining and talking about multi-professional working is to over-simplify.

Øvretveit (1993, cited in Pearson and Spencer 1997) defines a community multi-disciplinary team as a

> ... small group of people, usually from different professions and agencies, who relate to each other to contribute to the common goal of meeting the health and social needs of one client, or those of a client population in the community.

Payne (2000) suggests that multi-professional implies several different professional groups working together and multi-disciplinary refers to the knowledge and skills underlying particular professional roles. In the same text he describes inter-professional working requiring professionals to make adaptations to their roles in order to interact with roles of other professionals.

In defining teams and teamworking the World Health Organization (1984) definition is

> A group who share a common health goal and common objectives, determined by community needs, to the achievement of which each member of the team contributes, in accordance with his or her competencies and skill and in accordance with the function of others.

This would seem to be useful in the context of specialist palliative care.

The Calman and Hine Report (Department of Health 1995), which specifically talked about cancer services, together with the National Health Service (NHS) White Paper, The New NHS: Modern, Dependable (Department of Health 1997), focus attention on the need for high quality teamwork to provide a comprehensive and flexible service.

Teambuilding and building relationships in teams imply the need for cohesion and trust. They also suggest that team issues need to be worked on in order to get tasks completed. Organizations do not stay still and teams within them change as individual workers move on. The issue of conflict and collaboration will be examined more closely but it is vital that multi-professional teams can look both outward and inward. A team in conflict has often lost sight of its task and may jeopardize the need to co-operate with other agencies and groups of professionals. In this situation the patient's voice would be lost.

Payne (2000) suggests that managers and organizations often label groups of workers as a team in the hope that they wish they would, or hope they will, work together. The need to select team members who can work together will be examined later in the chapter.

The three professionals most commonly referred to as needing close working relationships in health and social care legislation are doctors, nurses and social workers. There are great differences in training, respon-sibilities and salaries. The values that underpin these professions and that will be examined later as providing a degree of conflict, differ in some vital ways. These professions have changed over time and their development needs to be understood because it has a part to play in the context of multi-professional working.

Developments in multi-professional working in hospitals and the community

Pietroni, in his 1994 paper on inter-professional teamwork, traces the his-tory of hospitals and their functioning, suggesting that 'groups of workers' coming together to care for patients began with the building of hospitals which were in medieval times run by religious and charitable bodies, much as hospices have developed in modern times.

Pietroni (1994) examined the bureaucratization of health and social care during the nineteenth century followed by what he described as the milita-rization of medical care following the Crimean, Boer and First World Wars. These early pioneers recognized that soldiers needed both physicians and nurses to meet their needs.

After the Second World War and the emergence of the Welfare State, the situation changed. The NHS had three structures, which we can still partly see today. The hospital run by the medical superintendent and matron, the general practitioners (GPs) who set up as self-employed practitioners and the community services headed by the Medical Officer of Health. Hospital and community team social workers specializing in child and adult physical and mental health were employed by the NHS and it was not until the

1970s, following the Seebohm Report (1968), that the majority of social work practitioners were employed by social services.

The problem for the modern social worker is the increasing use of workers as agents of social control. Complex legislation such as the Children Act (1989) and the NHS and Community Care Act (1990) define the role of social workers as assessors for service provision and risk, leading sometimes to criminal prosecution. This is a profession that was originally trained to act as therapist and supporter.

Nurses were originally seen as assistants to doctors, but during the 1970s and 1980s they demanded more autonomy. Project 2000 was to change nurse training to a more academic, college-based training with practical experience in hospital, not the other way round. In hospice and specialist palliative care teams nurses are by far the biggest professional group and hold most of the key managerial positions.

The Royal College of General Practitioners has been responsible for the development of GPs who were originally seen as secondary to hospital doctors. The last 30 years has seen the grouping of doctors and nurses in health centres.

The concept of group practices and the development of proper training for GPs has been a crucial community development. As a consequence of very recent reforms in the NHS there are now larger groupings of GPs with expanded budgetary powers. The primary care teams are key in the network of care for terminally ill people in the community, and specialist palliative care teams interface with these teams on a day-to-day basis. These teams often know the patient and family well before the specialists in palliative care become involved.

In the 1950s a typical general practice team consisted of one or two doctors with an administrator. Changes in the contractual arrangements over time led to the creation of new nursing posts and different professions attached to the practices. Payne (2000) identified that the current arrangement of purchaser/provider split demands co-operation and efficiency in health and that social care and professional/user partnerships provide the new context in which multi-professional teamwork has to function.

Multi-professionals working within the specialist context of palliative care

There is very little research material about the way multi-professional teams function in hospice and specialist palliative care teams. Hill (1998) studied the internal dynamics of multi-professional hospital palliative care teams by focused interviews of eight professionals working in several hospitals—three nurses, three doctors and two social workers—all had spent between 1 and 7 years working in the setting.

Hill (1998) identified the following benefits for the multi-professional: education, access to other health care professionals and support. The organizational culture was an important factor affecting team operation. The participants in this study felt that specialist palliative care was not well respected and suffered from marginalization from the rest of the hospital. It is not hard to see that this can lead to the need for specialist teams to become very close-knit units who could isolate themselves from the hospital culture. It has far-reaching implications for patients, clients and the drive to build the skills of specialist palliative care into the mainstream of the NHS. The opportunities to extend knowledge about pain and symptom control and the emphasis on holistic care, so central to palliative care, could be diminished.

Cowley *et al.* (2002) used a multiple case study design to explore the provision of palliative care and continuing care. The study demonstrated that an effective model of palliative care provision could be found where professional groups and organizations are able to capitalize on the differences in philosophy and culture of the different professional groups. Regular multidisciplinary meetings were described by one GP quoted in the study as being a contributory factor in enhancing good practice for patients by helping different professionals understand each other's role. The way different professionals would make sense of a patient's situation could also increase knowledge and skill. For example, anxiety as a symptom in a patient could be understood and addressed in a number of ways. The importance of thinking about the symptom and how to help would create the culture for shared learning. Bliss *et al.* (2000, cited in Cowley *et al.* 2002) stated

... that professionals cannot work independently to meet individuals' needs but must work within organisational policies and legislation as well as professional codes of practice and that inter-agency working plays an important part in effective palliative care.

Thus we are looking at small teams of different professional workers collaborating with each other and the possible difficulties that occur when collaborating across agency structures. Cowley *et al.* (2002) found that geographically dispersed and fragmented services had great difficulty in establishing co-ordinated services. They describe the circular relationship between inadequate resources, disputes about service responsibility and the breakdown of interpersonal relationships in areas where services were over-stretched; a familiar description to those of us working in the field. Cowley *et al.* (2002) quote a palliative care patient:

> I think I cope because of all the people that surround me … all give me different kinds of strengths … they are all very positive.

This quote from a satisfied palliative care patient demonstrates that multi-professional teams, when they work well, provide physical and emotional containment.

Firth (1997) describes another patient:

> Mary, age 56, who had only a few weeks to live, returned to the Day Hospice and poured out her distress, anger, longing for things to be different, her fear of what dying would be like and, later on, sadness at not seeing her grandchildren grow up. In a patients' discussion group she said that coming back to the hospice had been like crawling under a warm blanket that held her safe whilst she expressed her grief.

Cowley *et al.* (2002) make the connection between a multi-disciplinary palliative care service that is timely, needs led, responsive and innovative and the satisfaction of patients.

Conflict and collaboration

Language, communication, values, professional loyalty, role ambiguity and role blurring are flagged up as problems in teamworking by Payne (2000), Øvretveit *et al.* (1997), Hill (1998) and many others. Issues of power and inequality were identified as affecting decision making and policy development (Hill 1998).

A useful way of commencing the discussion about these issues is to look at what happens in terms of boundaries. Hornby (1993) suggests that a boundary is the defining limit of any system, in human terms, of any person, group of people or organisation. Although specialist palliative care services need boundaries in order to concentrate services and skills within a specialist grouping it can both help and hinder service users. Collaborative working requires us to work at the interface of a number of different boundaries, those between individuals and helpers, carers and workers, fellow workers, professionals, agencies and community groups (Hornby 1993).

At times boundaries between professional and patient are challenged when a professional worker is found to be terminally ill or bereaved. Generally there is a policy about engaging bereaved volunteers but it is not always recognized as a major issue when employing or continuing to employ staff.

Professional workers in palliative care settings are always making relationships with terminally ill patients and then preparing for the ending of
the relationships through death, so the interface of the boundary is even
more complex. The worker, the family and the patient can be caught up in
an immensely powerful emotional experience, which can often end suddenly. The worker begins or has already begun another cycle of professional relating. Powerful emotions can be released in the staff members, for
example, love, anger, respect, fear and anxiety. Often they are projected
onto other members of the team, the organization, the worker's own family
and sometimes the patient and their family. Attention to boundaries, both
professional and personal, is vital for the health of the individual and the
organization and the tasks it performs. Workers need a safe place to examine where their strong feelings are coming from.

Firth (2000) suggests that psychoanalytic concepts of fragmentation
and integration, which characterise the inner world of individuals, are a
helpful way of thinking about institutional processes as the institutional
boundary struggles to contain the primitive anxieties of patients and workers facing life and death issues on a daily basis. Splitting, denigration and
scapegoating of staff members of different professions and of outside agencies are identified as ways of maintaining a sense of well-being within an
institution when the individuals are under great stress.

> The hospice social worker visited the hospital ward where a young man was
> dying of lung cancer. The patient and family struggled to understand the
> sudden onset of his disease. The patient blamed his occupation and his
> family agreed with him but told the social worker that they thought smoking
> had caused his cancer. They were furious with him and doubted their ability
> to care for him at home. The hospital staff wanted his bed and became angry
> with the family for not taking him home and being responsible.

In this example feelings such as fear, anxiety, blame and obligation
needed a place to be safely explored with the patient and family. Sometimes
if issues such as these are not addressed with the patient and family they
can be projected onto the professional carers. In this case the hospital staff
demanded a hospice bed only to be told there was no vacancy, leading to
anger at the hospice staff who managed the resources.

Obholzer and Roberts (1994) describe how work settings in the helping
professions affect workers and how collective or institutional defences
determine organization structures and practices. They reflect that society
also has contradictory attitudes to nurses and doctors, on the one hand ide-
alization and on the other blame and responsibility. As far as social workers
are concerned the attitudes are less mixed. Social workers in general are

'damned if they do' or 'damned if they don't'. Specialist palliative care social work provides a setting where society's impossible task is somewhat less obvious. A very important paper, which examined institutional defences and nursing tasks, was written by Menzies (1960). It was the result of an extensive consultancy by Menzies and describes how the system of tasks carried out by nurses, and their lack of an opportunity to reflect on interactions with patients, led to denial and avoidance in relating to patients.

Forty years on nurses, doctors and social workers spend a great deal of time completing forms, that is, recording and auditing their work, all of which detracts from spending time with patients and their families. The need for record keeping and audit must be balanced with the need to keep patient centered.

We will see later how the concept of reflective practice, identified by Menzies, was later taken up by Schon (1987) and Pietroni (1991) in multi-professional education.

Institutional development

Institutions like families and individuals have life cycle transitions. Hospices have usually been formed by small groups of idealistic individuals. The common sense of purpose holds the team together and by necessity team members, whether professionals or volunteers, have many different roles. Success brings the need for more structure and management. Ajemian (1995) identifies this stage as being characterized by a lack of self-care amongst team members where personal limits (boundaries) are not acknowledged. This is closely followed by the need for formal programmes and an increasing definition of role and professional management, sometimes resented by founders of hospices.

Ajemian (1995) sees the tension as being between patient and family need, a firm financial base and future planning, that is, between idealism and pragmatism. If these stages can be negotiated successfully then roles are better understood and delineated. Professional expertise and additional staff and services are usually required as the hospice or specialist palliative care team balances idealistic humanistic concerns with a pragmatic response to legal and financial pressures from the community and society.

What about role and role ambiguity?

There is little doubt that workers in hospice and palliative care settings should have plenty of non-specialized professional work experience before joining the team. Ajemian (1995) identifies the need for staff to have a strong professional identity before recruitment because of the need to be secure enough within their professional role to allow other staff to sometimes share some aspects of it without being threatened. A number of workers have identified that the role of the clinical nurse specialist or Macmillan nurse overlaps most with medical and social work roles.

A rational, intellectual view would be to suggest that there is enough work to go round but if workers are feeling devalued or stressed then the overlapping of roles can cause conflict. Where the Macmillan nurses are employed by one agency, the doctors by the hospice and the social worker by social services, making connections and sorting out conflicts requires time and trust.

In palliative care with its commitment to holistic care the task is not always easy to define. The recognition of multiple needs and quality of life considerations requires a multi-professional approach and patients and families can choose who they talk to when they come into contact with different team members because palliative care is less fragmented. Sometimes this can lead to role confusion and conflict. The case for good clinical supervision, both internally and externally, is clearly made by these considerations. There is also a need for education in communication skills and loss and bereavement across disciplines in hospices. We have seen how medicine, nursing and social work have developed over the last hundred years and it is not difficult to see how the historical development has affected the way the different professions view and value each other. Both social work and nursing have a largely female workforce, whilst medicine has been traditionally a male occupation. Clearly training and levels of responsibility play a part but the gender issues may have also contributed to unequal pay, which can cause conflicts between team members.

Hill (1998) identified issues of power and inequality in specialist palliative care teams and pointed out that despite declaring that they favour a consensual approach, in practice they follow the traditional model of working, that is, accepting a medical lead. They tended to attribute conflict in the team as personality clashes. In palliative care the doctor still bears ultimate medico-legal responsibility but this is now shared much more by other professionals.

In hospices there is a strong argument for case management and clinical supervision to be split particularly where the team is working with complex family issues. A case manager would take responsibility for the way the multi-professional team worked together to meet the needs of the family as a whole. The clinical supervisor role would focus on the individual professional's clinical practice. Overall case management could check that family conflicts were not affecting the professional team performance and vice versa.

A young mother disclosed to a hospice nurse that her husband had sexually abused her young child. Her concern was that when she died this would continue. The nurse felt this was a secret she had been given and could not divulge to the team. Another member of the hospice team noticed the husband's behaviour towards his 8-year-old daughter and expressed her concern to the hospice social worker who felt enormous concern for the child. The social worker had a duty to investigate because of the Children Act (1989), the importance of protecting vulnerable children and her ethical and value base as a professional social worker. The young mother was by this time very ill and found communicating difficult. She told the social worker that the hospice nurse knew all about it. The hospice nurse felt she was duty bound by her professional code of ethics not to talk to the social worker. Clearly the question of risk overrode these issues. The issue was resolved but not without some acrimony. The positive outcome was a training programme for hospice staff around child protection issues and an identified need for another professional to act as overall case manager. The child's position was thoroughly examined and her maternal grandmother became her carer after the death of her mother.

In this case example we can see the conflict being based on different professional values and a lack of knowledge about collective responsibility. However, when workers are under stress they often go back to stereotyping other professionals, for example, the arrogant doctor, the bossy nurse or the left-wing social worker.

If we look at this example from the patient, her husband and child's view, their voices were eventually heard but it could have been very different if the workers had not resolved their differences and had lost sight of the task. The young mother desperately wanted her daughter to be safe after her death. She told the nurse because she wanted some action. The husband did not say he wanted help with his relationship with his daughter but he behaved in such a way that demonstrated the problem.

Confidentiality issues frequently surface as areas of conflict. A well run multi-disciplinary meeting can provide a forum for team members to consider such questions as 'Who does information belong to?', 'When does risk override patient autonomy?' and so on. Such a meeting can help teams develop and reflect on their practice whilst allowing for differing professional perspectives in considering the patients' needs. Although specialist palliative care professionals share many of the same values and a commitment to holistic care, subtle differences in value base can be a problem.

The need for research in this area is evident and would help to identify what the formal rules and shared meanings are which help to contribute to the code of ethics of each profession. For example, in social work, values reflect a great deal of recent writing and research concerning oppression and discrimination. More important is the need to identify the informal rules and meanings that derive from sub-cultures in organizations.

Inter-group relating in specialist palliative care teams and hospices can often be conflictual because individual professional members have a problem about managing dual membership, that of doctor, nurse, social worker, psychologist, occupational therapist or physiotherapist and member of a multi-professional team.

Firth (2000) talks about staff groups, led by outside consultants, being a place for reflection, connection and attendance to personal issues raised by the work. However, she points out that the task must be the focus.

Finally, the issue of reflection and reflective practice is crucial in palliative care as in all forms of health and social care. Pietroni (1995) points out that Schon (1987) examined the relationship between the individual professionals and their organizational task. His ideas about a double feedback loop of action, reflection and learning, addresses the tension between theory generated by practice and theory applied to practice. Firth (2000) suggests that different professionals collaborating in palliative care can be helped towards reflective practice by attending small groups of multi-professionals. Currently, clinical supervision aimed at reflective practice tends to take place in single professional groups. Schon (1987) talks about the need to develop a form of professional artistry, which is stimulated by living connections between theory, intuition and practice. A small group setting would be ideal, providing it is led by an experienced group practitioner who is committed to multi-professional working.

The issue of recruitment based on maturity, personality and professional qualification is an important one, but also we see the need to appoint workers who can co-operate with other disciplines. Many workers argue that inter-professional education can lead to more effective inter-professional teamworking and these issues have been addressed elsewhere in this book, together with the involvement of service users in some of these educational initiatives.

Increasing the involvement of patients and carers in multi-professional teams

We have seen that people expect more from health and social services. Advocacy services for traditionally less articulate groups, for example, children in care, the homeless and people with a mental health or learning disability are now widely accepted. The explosion in information technology has contributed to give all sections of the community more access to information about health and social issues.

In palliative care, patients and families facing a terminal illness can access a wide range of written and electronic information about diagnosis and treatment. Often they become more knowledgeable about their disease than their GP and this will clearly affect the relationship between the two. The boundary and power issues identified earlier will be changed. One of the commonest feelings expressed by palliative care patients and their families is powerlessness. Changing this by giving clearly understood information about illness and treatment should be seen as central.

A common complaint for health and social care professionals is that dealing with endless questions from patients and clients takes time. These professionals might see some families and patients who complain as a huge problem rather than joining in partnership with them. Different team members may view things differently.

> A middle-aged woman living alone was dying of liver cancer. On a visit to see a consultant, she felt that her fears and questions were brushed aside. During a regular visit by the social worker from the hospice the patient asked for help in writing a letter of complaint. The letter was written and the consultant considered its contents and then arranged another consultation for the patient. In the meantime, the hospice nurses who heard about the letter and held the consultant in high regard were furious with the social worker.

In this example one of the learning points was that of the role of advocacy, which the hospice team had not really explored before, although it had been raised previously. The social worker realized that the communication issues between the hospice team and himself were also part of the problem. Was he using the situation to 'have a go' at his medical colleagues, identifying as a marginalized member of the team with the weak and disempowered patient? In palliative care the unconscious needs for all professions to rescue are particularly powerful when faced with the powerlessness engendered by cancer and its treatments.

Øvretveit et al. (1997) states that client involvement can mean one of four things: consulting them, information-giving about what has been decided, jointly deciding or the person decides or does something themselves. He explains that these four things can operate differently throughout the journey of illness, and at the level of service operations, for example, information about a change in opening times of an out-patient clinic or at a strategic planning stage, for example, consulting people about service planning.

In the example above, the patient had been given information about her condition; her complaint was the manner in which it was given. She felt depersonalized and worthless. Standard setting around information-giving needs to include auditing the way it is presented interpersonally.

Information needs to be given in understandable forms. A group of elderly Asian women with very little 'English' felt disempowered by the hospital setting in which their husbands died. Moreover, they had no access to specialist bereavement care but there was a suitable service in a nearby town. The notices in the hospital advertising the service were in their spoken language but as with many older people from their district of Pakistan they could not read or write.

McLeod and Bywaters (2000) draw attention to the unnecessary suffering of many people in the course of life-threatening illness and this is despite the best efforts of professionals in health care generally. They refer to the lack of impact specialist palliative care has had on other parts of the health service. They point out that, as yet, there is no self-directed, unified and recognized social movement spanning life-threatening illness parallel to that of the disability rights movement, but they identify the preliminary elements of collective self-organization, particularly with regard to gay HIV/AIDS initiatives. Hospice-based social work is seeking the views of service users in order to influence future provision in a project called 'Involve: What service users want from specialist palliative care social work' (West 2000). This UK development project is being advised by academics, practitioners and service users and is supported by the Joseph Rowntree Foundation.

This brings into focus the need for hospices and specialist palliative care units to be systematic in the way in which they involve patients in decision making and partnerships. They need to consider carefully what the effects will be of seeking the views of patients and families and all the professionals involved. For example, it is important that the involvement should be purposeful.

> Service users in one hospice were asked to consider a change of provision only to find that the decision had already been made at a senior management level. This led to professionals and patients feeling angry, demoralized and worthless.

One area that patients and carers complain about is having to keep telling their story to different members of the team. Confidentiality policies are often introduced without a multi-professional discussion. For example, teams need to consider how information is stored and recorded and the benefits of keeping a single file or of different departments of the service maintaining their own notes. This is one area that could be focused on and would provide useful information about professional perceptions and assessments. Jones and McIntyre (2002) report the outcome of implementing multi-disciplinary notes in a specialist palliative care unit and conclude that care was becoming more directly patient focused because of the presence of multi-disciplinary care plans at the bedside. In order to review or assess patient care, professionals had to approach the bedside. The team learnt to be honest about each other's documentation and acknowledged that clinical governance and clinical effectiveness needed documentation to be accurate. It also led to more discussions about role and values.

Øvretveit et al. (1997) discuss the way changes in patient or client power have affected their relationship with professionals and, in turn, how it affects the way professionals relate to each other, for example, professionals are more ready to challenge each other. He suggests that these changes produce an equalizing effect that undermines traditional power relations in multi-professional teams.

Giving patients a voice means we must look at power issues. Payne (2000) suggests that as well as power being seen as being oppressive to certain groups and professionals, it can be used positively. He defines power as being 'getting what we want'. His example of involving users of services in their own care planning means making explicit the influence they can have and the practices and procedures which give them rights, and the fact that they are experts in their own problems.

In multi-professional teams, doctors are often seen as having over-riding expert power. Payne (2000) suggests that this imposes unnecessary burdens on them by referring inappropriate things to them. A dying patient may only listen to the hospice consultant or they may avoid the doctor and only talk to the chaplain. Payne (2000) concludes that power is a matter of perception and relationship.

Some hospices have already included patients in the hospice organization by involving them as trustees. Clearly the problem of continuity in involving ill people in strategic planning has to be addressed.

Conclusions

In specialist palliative care the emphasis on holistic care means that a range of skills are required to be able to intervene in the physical, psychosocial and spiritual needs of patients and families. The multi-professional team brings together individuals with a diversity of training to share the goal of improving the quality of life of the patient.

The context in which hospices and specialist palliative care teams function has changed dramatically in the last 20 years as people expect more from services and are given a voice about their care. User involvement, and professional/user partnerships do already influence multi-professional working. Over the next 10 years it will be interesting to see how patients can further influence care provision. Will the challenge to make palliative care more widely available be met and where will the drive for this come from?

Multi-professional teams have to communicate and collaborate within their own agencies and across agencies. We have looked at some of the areas of difficulty and at the positives for both patient and team member, but we need more research in this area.

How will inter-professional education impact upon collaborative working? There are clearly established needs for communication skills training for all professionals.

Walters (2002) states that death and loss, like birth, are natural processes and workers in these fields are therefore akin to midwives. The dying or bereaved are making a highly personal pilgrimage and the professional caregiver walks with them some of the way.

The patient centrality of this model challenges the multi-professional team to work in more integrated ways. In the same article Walters poses the question whether, or how far, each professional can walk with each patient.

Team members need each other. Recognizing each other's professional and personal strengths and weaknesses is essential to provide services that recognize the uniqueness of the individual and their family and that care must involve the whole team.

Oliviere et al. (1998) quote the practice example of Louis, aged 42, who has a brain tumour with extensive secondaries. All the counselling available did not have a positive effect on the pain. Alternatively, no amount of morphine or other analgesia blotted out the marital conflict and financial problems he, his wife and two children were experiencing as a result of a failing business and his mood swings. The various aspects of this person's life had to be understood and worked with as a whole.

References

Ajemian, I. (1995) *The Inter-disciplinary Team*. In: Doyle, D., Hanks, G. and MacDonald, N. (ed.) *Oxford Textbook of Palliative Medicine*, pp. 17–27. Oxford: Oxford University Press.

Cowley, S., Bliss, J., Matthew, A. and McVey, G. (2002) Effective inter-agency and inter-professional working: facilitators and barriers. *International Journal of Palliative Nursing* 8, 30–9.

Department of Health (1995) *A Policy Framework for Commissioning Cancer Services* (The Calman–Hine Report). London: Department of Health.

Department of Health (1997) *The New NHS: Modern, Dependable* (HMSO CM 3807). London: The Stationery Office.

Firth, P. (1997) Understanding bereavement. *Connect* 3, pp. 6–7.

Firth, P. (2000) Picking up the pieces: groupwork in palliative care. In: Manor, O. (ed.) *Ripples: Groupwork in Different Settings*, pp. 16–31. London: Whiting & Birch.

Hill, A. (1998) Multi-professional teamwork in a hospital palliative care team. *International Journal of Palliative Nursing* 4, 214–21.

Hornby, S. (1993) *Collaborative Care: Interprofessional, Interagency and Interpersonal.* Oxford: Blackwell.

Jones, K. and McIntyre, M. (2002) A multi-disciplinary approach to terminal care. *European Journal of Palliative Care* 9, 21–4.

McLeod, E. and Bywaters, P. (2000) *Social Work, Health and Equality.* London: Routledge.

Menzies, I.E.P. (1960) Social systems as a defence against anxiety: an empirical study of the nursing service of a general hospital. In: Trist, E. and Murray, H. (ed.) *The Social Engagement of Social Science, Volume I: The Socio-Psychological Perspective*, pp. 439–62. London: Free Association Books.

Obholzer, A. and Roberts, V.Z. (ed.) (1994) *The Unconscious at Work.* London: Routledge.

Oliviere, D., Hargreaves, R. and Monroe, B. (1998) *Good Practices in Palliative Care.* Aldershot: Ashgate.

Øvretveit, J., Matthias, P. and Thompson, T. (ed.) (1997) *Interprofessional Working for Health and Social Care.* Basingstoke: Palgrave.

Payne, M. (2000) *Teamwork in Multi-professional Care.* Basingstoke: Palgrave.

Pearson, P. and Spencer, J. (1997) *Promoting Teamwork in Primary Care— A Research Based Approach.* London: Arnold.

Pietroni, M. (1991) (ed.) *Right or Privilege?* London: Central Council for Education and Training in Social Work.

Pietroni, P. (1994) Inter-professional teamwork. In: Leathard, A. (ed.) *Going Inter-professional: Working Together for Health and Welfare*, pp. 77–89. London: Routledge.

Pietroni, M. (1995) The nature and aims of professional education for social workers. In: Yelloly, M. and Hentel, M. (ed.) *Learning and Teaching in Social Work*, pp. 34–50. London: Jessica Kingsley.

Schon, D. (1987) *Educating the Reflective Practitioner.* London: Jossey Bass.

Walters, T. (2002) Spirituality in palliative care: opportunity or burden. *Palliative Medicine* 16, 133–9.

West, A. (2000) What service users want from specialist palliative care social work. *Hospice Bulletin* May, 8(1), 3–4.

World Health Organization (1984) *Glossary of Terms used in the 'Health for All' Series No. 1–8.* Geneva: World Health Organization.

9

Palliative medicine

James Gilbert

Introduction

It may be less true now than when said to Dame Cicely Saunders in 1951 that 'it's the doctors who desert the dying' (Barrett 1951). But even today, of the professions key to palliative care provision, it is generally not doctors who enjoy the reputation of being the most patient centred. The truth is that being patient focused does not come naturally to all doctors. In this chapter I shall identify and explore some of the reasons for this before analysing some of the assumptions underlying the idea of 'a voice for the voiceless'. Some reflections on advocacy follow and I conclude with an examination of ways in which our own values have an important role in the delivery of satisfactory palliative care.

How not to be patient focused

Before considering morally justifiable ways of not being patient focused, it seems important to acknowledge that there are times when most, if not all, healthcare professionals fall short as a result of being either insufficiently caring or insufficiently competent. While neither of these two deficiencies can be avoided altogether, all healthcare professionals have a duty to minimize their impact on good practice. In doing so we need to achieve clarity about the limits of our professional competence as well as making a commitment to life-long learning in order to maintain and develop that competence. Recent changes to the way in which doctors are trained may bode well for the future with a greater emphasis now being placed on developing communication skills, reflective practice, healthcare ethics and problem-based learning. These or other ways need to be found for preserving the highly caring attitudes evident in the early careers of most healthcare professionals. Specific efforts towards nurturing our compassion may help (Sogyal Rinpoche 1993) and, on a more prosaic level, guarding against over commitment and over work wherever possible.

Focus on disease

To refer to 'the heart attack in bed three' is an example of being exclusively disease focused and is unlikely ever to be morally justifiable. There are however many occasions on which the medical needs of patients will be best met by a doctor whose primary focus is on the disease and its effects. Consider, for instance, a single mother called Carol who has metastatic breast cancer. If Carol were to experience increasing back pain and begin to feel unsteady on her feet she would be at high risk of spinal cord compression. In this situation if her doctor was not primarily disease focused Carol might, within 24 hours, have lost irrevocably her ability to walk. Of course such situations are not the norm for most doctors but the need always to be alert to circumstances of reversible physical deterioration should be a key part of the practice of all doctors. The retention of a disease focus alongside, but not dominating, a patient focus is likely to benefit Carol in a number of other ways. It is probable that Carol will need information about her likely prognosis, both in terms of time and of the ways in which her disease may progress (Christakis 1999). While the sensitive exploration of whether and when Carol may need this information requires a patient focus, the validity of the information itself will require careful focus on the nature of the disease. The challenge for different doctors at different times is to use their technical knowledge for the benefit of the individual patient. For the pathologist reviewing the histological specimen the focus—both literally and metaphorically—needs to be on disease, in the expectation that the results will be used in the context of the individual patient. For the general practitioner visiting the person with advanced illness at home an individual patient focus in the context of their family will primarily be required.

Focus on research

The practice of modern healthcare is built on reliable knowledge identified by those who have gone before. Many, if not most, doctors recognize a moral obligation to add where possible to the sum of reliable knowledge in order that healthcare can improve in the future. To do so requires a research focus that may at times impinge on an ability to be patient focused. Although the moral justification for research seems clear, the possibility of this focus impinging on patient centredness is worrying. Specifically to use people today purely as a means by which knowledge is advanced, albeit for the benefit of others in the future, is morally unjustified (Kant 1964). It is the open explanation and unpressurized invitation for today's patient to participate, or not, in research that is supposed to provide the necessary safeguard. The extent to which such safeguards are effective in practice is sometimes limited and we should acknowledge that some research leads more reliably to career enhancement for the researcher than to improved patient care. While not themselves entirely benign, the methods of qualitative research do offer genuine opportunities to gain greater understanding of the lived patient experience.

Paternalism

To be paternalistic involves both forming a judgement about what's best for another individual and then seeking to impose that judgement (Boyd *et al.* 1997). Perfectly appropriate for small children and probably enacted as often by mothers as fathers, so perhaps a shame that the term parentalism is in less common usage! For adult patients, it seems clear that paternalism jeopardizes patient centredness, affording as it does insufficient respect to the autonomy of the individual. Of course patients are entitled to seek—and to receive (Fallowfield 2001)—the guidance of their doctor about what might be best for them. This willingness on the part of the patient removes one of the two required elements for paternalism and returns the encounter to a patient centred one. The attempted imposition on a patient of the action perceived as best is likely to be based on an excessively disease-focused attitude. For example, mild anaemia in a patient weakened by advanced cancer may at times be best responded to by explanation and encouraging acceptance rather than admission to hospital or hospice for blood transfusion. A subtle form of paternalism may be exhibited by the doctor who exaggerates the benefits of transfusion rather than pursuing a potentially upsetting discussion about how little medical intervention might truly have to offer. Equally a nihilistic attitude is a particular risk in palliative medicine and may at times also underlie paternalistic behaviours.

Focus on the institution

I have sought to consider various ways in which the focus of healthcare professionals may at times not be on the patient, and sometimes justifiably so. Of these, paternalism, focus on disease and focus on research are particularly, if not exclusively, behaviours of doctors. Focusing on the institution, rather than on the patient, is a concern for doctors but at least as much so for other healthcare professionals.

The most prominent institution for palliative care professionals is the hospice. Central to the philosophy of the hospice movement is recognizing and valuing the individuality of patients and those close to them. Yet we should be aware of some ways in which healthcare professionals may be limited in their ability to be patient centred by a focus on the institution. Douglas (1992) painted a particularly bleak picture of the hospice movement charging it in particular with unjustifiable separateness and selectivity amounting to 'the singling out of a precious few for deluxe dying'. But even 10 years on, his challenge should not be lightly dismissed. At any one time most people with palliative care needs will be at home, many will be in hospital and a particularly vulnerable group will be in nursing or residential homes. The need therefore is paramount for hospices to be inclusive, accessible and welcoming to the widest variety of people. Where, as is commonly the case in the UK, hospices have contracts or service agreements to provide specialist palliative care for defined populations this need may indeed be a statutory obligation. In order to meet this obligation, among other requirements

◆ the buildings must be provided in the locations best suited to the users rather than determined by history or what best suits trustees, staff or volunteers;

◆ admissions policies should reflect the meeting of palliative care need, rather than being based on diagnosis (often of cancer);

◆ openness to people of all faiths, and of none, must be an inclusive reality rather than a slogan.

I should make clear that although a focus on the institution will compete at times with attempts to be patient focused, I am not suggesting that we abandon shared professional values, of which more later in the chapter.

A voice for the voiceless—underlying assumptions

Various assumptions underlie the idea of 'a voice for the voiceless', most obviously perhaps a need for advocacy—literally, speaking for another. The requirements for legitimate advocacy are discussed later in the chapter, but first how can we be sure when people are truly voiceless? Of course when unconscious or having lost, through injury or illness, the capacity to think or communicate thought, patients can truly be said to be voiceless. Much more often, however, a much lesser degree of impairment may be evident and the term voicelessness is used to exaggerate the position of dis-advantaged patients experiencing a significant power imbalance between them and their healthcare professionals. It seems clear that, if not actually voiceless, patients *are* often disadvantaged and that power imbalances are real. A frightened and ill person confronted by a complicated and threat-ening diagnosis is obviously in a dependent position when consulting an expert healthcare professional. One might usefully note along the way that such power imbalances may be as important between patient and family as between patient and professional and that power imbalances also exist between healthcare professionals.

Recognition of the patient's disadvantaged position is increasingly explicit and various initiatives seek to compensate for this (National Health Service Executive 1999, Our Healthier Nation 2001). However, *assuming* a need for advocacy is dangerous and may paradoxically serve to empower the professionals who claim it, rather than the patient, and to diminish the trust and respect required for effective interprofessional team working. It may be further assumed that the values of healthcare professionals should be suppressed in order to give primacy to patient centredness. I shall argue that this latter is a misguided assumption and that our values as healthcare professionals are not only valid but that they form a fundamental part of what we ought to offer to patients, but not seek to impose upon them.

In summary, we do have a moral duty to identify those occasions when disadvantage to patients is so great as to amount to voicelessness and to recognize when advocacy is needed, but more commonly to realize when disadvantage is present but not so great as to amount to voicelessness. In these circumstances we could often more usefully concentrate on helping patients speak more effectively for themselves.

Legitimate advocacy

Acting as a patient's advocate is not easy, not least because healthcare colleagues do not always welcome such a role. Here power imbalances between healthcare professionals may add to difficulties. There may be times however when any lack of welcome is entirely justified and so we should consider carefully when advocacy *is* legitimate.

Firstly, a need for advocacy must be established. When patients are quite capable of speaking for themselves, even if they need help in doing so, a need for advocacy is not established.

Secondly, the desire for someone to act as advocate must be established. Even if an advocate is needed it must not be assumed that the patient desires it. Paradoxically, to do so would be an act of paternalism entailing a judgement as to what's best (that the patient should have an advocate) followed by an imposition on the patient without their consent.

Thirdly, it must be determined who should act as advocate in the circumstances concerned. This choice is of course the patient's, from among those able to act in this way. It should be remembered that patients may, confusingly, choose different healthcare professionals at different times to speak for them and may not be consistent in their wishes.

If these conditions for legitimate advocacy are met, and only if they are met, the courage then needs to be found to risk unpopularity with colleagues in speaking for the patient. The possibility of being respected by those colleagues is likely to be much increased if they have confidence that care has been taken to establish a role as legitimate advocate.

To be truly patient centred must we deny our own values?

Circumstances in which the values and beliefs of patients, those close to them and the healthcare professionals involved all coincide (Oliviere 2001) may still require much skilled and committed palliative care work but are not likely to challenge our patient centredness. One might therefore suppose that the more the values and beliefs of the healthcare professional are suppressed or even excluded the more patient centredness is safeguarded. I want to suggest however that the price for such a safeguard may be too high even if possible to achieve—which like Savulescu (Savulescu 1995) I doubt. Let me first be clear that there are times when suppressing the expression of our own values as healthcare professionals is entirely right. It seems obvious, for example, that for a hospice social worker who happens to be vegetarian to engage a disinterested patient in a discussion about the evils of meat eating would be wrong, as it would be for me to comment adversely on a patient's lack of concern for the progress of the England football team. More seriously, but similarly, as I have argued earlier the spiritual or religious beliefs of the healthcare professional should not be allowed to jeopardize patient centred care.

There are however some values and beliefs that differ importantly from these examples of individual values or values particular to the healthcare professional concerned. Where, in distinction, values are *shared* among healthcare professionals, to an extent that makes those values integral to the type of healthcare concerned, the suppression of those values may do more harm than good. The clearest example for palliative care is that of acceptance of dying as an inevitable and normal part of life. To return to the example of Carol, were she to seek the support of her homecare nurse to bolster her belief that her teenage children should not be told of her advancing disease, an important conflict of values might result. The homecare nurse, regarding dying as a normal and inevitable part of living, is likely to recognize through reflection and experience that openness with children in such a situation both better honours our duty to tell the truth and results in less long-term distress. And yet the patient centred approach on the face of it suggests a different course of action. Similarly for the nurse in an in-patient unit looking after Carol in her last week or so of life might wish to decline to give repeated vigorous and intrusive enemas even at Carol's own request because of a soundly based conviction that more harm than good would result. I am not suggesting in either instance that the skilled and compassionate palliative care worker would seek confrontation or argument, but that the exercising of good professional judgement may need to be based on appropriate shared professional values, and that it may on occasion be more important to safeguard those values than to be maximally patient focused. Specific to the doctor's role, there will be occasions when declining to do harm to someone with widespread and advanced cancer by attempting cardio-pulmonary resuscitation will be judged (rightly, I suggest) as more important than acceding to the apparent wishes of that person.

Of course for particular patients even very close to the ends of their lives the palliative care approach may not be acceptable. Helping such patients find alternative styles of healthcare may be the most important duty of the healthcare professional when basic values integral to palliative care are rejected. Equally important is the making explicit of these values in both internationally agreed definitions (World Health Organization 1990) and local service provider information. Where professional judgement is an expectation of patients and those close to them there is a duty to make and communicate that judgement on the basis of shared and explicit professional values. In order not to fall into the trap of paternalism any guidance towards a particular action for the benefit of the patient must stop short of coercion involving either threat or misinformation.

Hopper (2000) suggests that 'the life of a professional is essentially a matter of reconciling competing values and choosing the higher "good" for each individual'. Providing these values are never imposed and are shared, explicit and professionally rather than personally based, I agree with her.

Conclusion

Being patient focused is easy to claim and sometimes difficult to do. I have argued that attention needs to be given to distinguish when a patient focus is crucial from times when a different focus is required. In examining underlying assumptions some of the pitfalls of being too ready to take on a role as patient's advocate have been identified and discussed. Finally, I have suggested that aiming to exclude any effect produced by our own values is not only likely to prove impossible to achieve but also may result in inadequate professional judgement. Circumstances have been described in which holding onto explicit, shared, professional values is likely to help rather than hinder us in making a valid contribution to patient care. If in the name of patient centredness we over react to the wrongs of paternalism we risk retreating to a role as disengaged 'technicians plus information providers'. This would amount to a failure of professional duty.

References

Barrett WR (1951) Personal communication to Cicely Saunders.

Boyd KM, Higgs R and Pinching AJ (1997) *The New Dictionary of Medical Ethics.* BMJ Publishing Group, London.

Christakis NA (1999) *Death Foretold: Prophecy and Prognosis in Medical Care.* University of Chicago Press, Chicago.

Douglas C (1992) For all the saints. *British Medical Journal,* 304:579.

Fallowfield L (2001) Participation of patients in decisions about treatment for cancer. *British Medical Journal,* 323:1144.

Hopper A (2000) Meeting the spiritual needs of patients through holistic practice. *European Journal of Palliative Care,* 7:60–2.

Kant I (1964) *Groundwork of the Metaphysic of Morals.* Patron HJ (trans). Harper and Row, New York.

National Health Service Executive (1999) *Patient and Public Involvement in the New NHS.* The Stationery Office, London.

Oliviere D (2001). User involvement in palliative care services. *European Journal of Palliative Care,* 8:238–41.

Our Healthier Nation (2001) The expert patient—a new approach to chronic disease management for the 21st Century. People and communities section of Our Healthier Nation website—http://www.ohn.gov.uk.

Savulescu J (1995) Rational non-interventional paternalism: Why doctors ought to make judgements of what is best for their patients. *Journal of Medical Ethics,* 21:327–31.

Sogyal Rinpoche (1993) *The Tibetan Book of Living and Dying.* Harper Collins, San Francisco.

World Health Organization (1990) *Cancer Pain Relief and Palliative Care.* Technical Report Series 804. World Health Organization, Geneva.

10

Palliative nursing

Mandy Stratford

Introduction

Palliative nursing commences from the moment that the patient and family are told that the disease is no longer responsive to curative treatment. Throughout the course of the illness they will come into close contact with nurses in various settings, so it is clear that palliative nursing is the responsibility of all nurses. Nurses have a privileged opportunity to influence the patient's experience. Using the supportive care model suggested by Davies and Oberle (1990) and examples from practice, the author shows how nurses in all care settings can remain patient focused and how nurses and the environment in which they work facilitate or obstruct patient and family involvement in care.

Role of the nurse

Several authors have attempted to define the role of the nurse in palliative care. These mainly descriptive accounts differ according to the setting in which the study took place; to date there is no clear agreement on a definition of palliative nursing. Most nurses in the UK would accept that their function is to assess the holistic needs of the patient and family and involve them in planning and evaluating appropriate interventions. The aim is to improve the quality of life and enable a dignified death (Lugton and Kindlen 1999). However, this does not capture the essence of palliative nursing, which lies in the nurse–patient relationship (Morse 1991). This is emphasized in the framework for specialist practice in palliative care proposed by Davies and Oberle (1990), which is widely recognized as the model for palliative nursing throughout the UK. The model describes six interwoven but discrete aspects of the nurse's role: valuing, connecting, empowering, finding meaning, doing for and preserving integrity.

Valuing

According to Davies and Oberle (1990), valuing has two components, global and particular. Global valuing is having respect for others regardless of the particular characteristics of an individual. This is a requirement of all nurses in the UK as the code for professional conduct (Nursing and Midwifery Council, 2002) clearly states, 'as a nurse or midwife you must respect the patient or client as an individual.' Furthermore, 'you are personally accountable for ensuring that you promote and protect the interests and dignity of patients and clients, irrespective of gender, age, race, ability, sexuality, economic status, lifestyle, culture and religious or political beliefs.'

Particular valuing is more individualized and develops after the nurse gets to know the patient. Nurses develop an understanding of the individual's unique characteristics and abilities, respecting the person for who they are. This important aspect of care needs continuous attention. It requires astute self-awareness of thoughts, attitudes and prejudices, as these could influence the nurse's approach to the patient. Patients who appear uncomplaining, who smile and look nice, who are able to communicate well and who are grateful and compliant tend to receive more time, contact and interested attention from nurses. By contrast, the unpopular patient who is demanding, heavily dependent, complains, is not grateful, has unsociable habits, does not comply, looks unkempt and is not able or does not wish to communicate, receives less attention, contact and time from nurses. The ability to recognize the reason for certain behaviours and to learn to value and respond to individual qualities will prevent the nurse from falling into the trap of labelling or categorizing the patient.

Connecting

Often it is the first point of contact between the nurse and the patient and family that makes the greatest impact as the following comments from a letter written by the family of a patient demonstrates.

> We were very scared about mum going to the hospice but we really shouldn't have been. Jo soon made us feel that this was the right place. From the minute we met her we knew that mum was safe. She took time to explain

things; showed us round the hospice and made us all feel like nothing was too much bother. Mum had a lot of confidence in her and that meant that we could relax a bit.

Davies and Oberle (1990) describe this initial contact as 'making the connection'. The nurse lays the foundation for an ongoing relationship to develop. In this example Jo, a staff nurse at the hospice, recognized the patient's and family's anxiety. By taking time to attend to their concerns and showing them around the unit and telling them how to access her, she established an immediate rapport with the patient and family.

Making the connection requires nurses to examine the manner in which they approach patients and families. A calm and unhurried approach and the ability to concentrate on only that person will be vital to the patient who may, up to this point, have felt they are just a number or a disease.

In their book, *The primacy of caring*, Benner and Wrubel (1989) stress the importance of spending time getting to know the person through the 'patient's story'. Nurses need to understand the impact of the illness, the human experience as well as the disease process, to provide appropriate nursing care. They need to know how the patient noticed their symptoms, what aspects of their life are affected and how the patient interprets this.

Davies and Oberle (1990) stress that connection will not occur until trust is established. In making the connection the focus is on what is most important to the patient and the family, yet many nursing procedures still reflect the agenda of the nurse or organization rather than that of the patient. For example, a nursing assessment seeks to obtain information about the patient and family on which to base nursing care. Some will be obtained at the time of admission but in palliative care, most will be gathered over time, when the patient feels comfortable about disclosing information that is more personal. However, nurses report feeling under increasing pressure to document as much information as possible at the time of admission. Reasons put forward include to meet legal and organizational requirements, such as risk management; to aid communication to a fragmented workforce; to demonstrate that they have discussed the subject with the patient; and the expectations of other team members (personal communications 2002). If nurses feel under pressure to meet these expectations, patient assessments become nursing assessments driven by the information needs of the nurse to prescribe care and document the impact of the disease rather than the illness. To deal with this from the patient perspective, Ellis (1999) proposes the use of a patient-centred model of assessment and documentation. However, such attempts are fruitless if there is little support from the organization to implement it, or if nurses and the wider team do not fully understand the importance this has for the delivery of patient-centred care.

To continue or 'sustain' the relationship, nurses must be available to spend time with the patient, share 'secrets' and give of themselves, as the following account demonstrates.

> Bill had been referred to the nurse specialist by his general practitioner (GP) for an assessment of his pain. He had been commenced on morphine by his GP, which had achieved excellent pain control. However, on collecting his repeat prescription three weeks later, he had noticed 'morphine' written on the box and had stopped taking it. He was now in considerable pain and refused any medication the GP offered. When I telephoned Bill he had seemed a bit hesitant but agreed to my visiting. His opening statement to me on the doorstep was, 'if you have come to tell me I have got to take that poison you can bugger off now'. When I replied that I was not there to do that but to see if I could offer any other suggestions that might be helpful and that would be acceptable to him, he invited me in. Initiating a conversation with Bill was hard work. I tried asking open questions in an attempt to assess the situation but he was very suspicious and seemed to be reluctant to engage in any way. His body language clearly indicated his defensiveness. I noticed a photograph on the television set in the centre of the room. It was of a war memorial. I thought that a bit unusual, so commented to Bill that I had noticed it had a prominent position in his home. Bill broke down in tears and went on to tell me that he had been on a warship during the Second World War. The ship had been bombed and he had been one of only a few survivors. He described how he had administered morphine injections to his friends from the supplies they each kept around their necks. He cried as he told me of the nightmares that still haunt him and how he continued to feel responsible for their deaths. He had not shared this with anyone else, not even his family.

> Over the following few weeks Bill and I talked more about his experience, morphine and the alternatives he might try. He seemed more open to my suggestions and when it came to the point where morphine was the most appropriate solution, he was willing to give it a try, knowing that he could always change his mind.

It is therefore of particular concern that the trend is for many clinical nurse specialists to work in a consultative capacity or short-term involvement with patients and families. Whilst the intention is to support and advise colleagues, as a role model, it undermines the most important and fundamental aspects of patient support and of the nurse's role in palliative care.

This component of connecting can be a great source of frustration for nurses with busy work schedules and those working in organizations that do not value or understand the need for this level of contact. However, it takes no longer to communicate well than badly. Quality time and the illusion of spending more time can be achieved if combined with other activities such as bathing or changing dressings. In a study of nurse–patient contact on in-patient units Dingman *et al.* (1999) found that nurses sitting and talking at the bedside for just 5 minutes increased patient satisfaction. Patients benefited psychologically from such action, felt reassured and had an increased sense of control and empowerment. In some settings, nurses have re-organized their work and break schedules to increase their contact with patients. For example, implementing audio-taped handovers in an in-patient unit enabled nurses on an early shift to spend an additional 45–60 minutes with patients that would previously have been spent on a verbal handover to colleagues. In another unit, the introduction of bedside handovers not only increased the time nurses spent in direct contact with the patient, but also enabled the patient to be actively involved in their care (author's own experience).

In developing close relationships, there is a risk that the patient feels abandoned or unsafe when, as they see it, their own nurse is not on duty. Nurses rarely work as lone practitioners; in palliative care they work as part of a much wider multidisciplinary team. It is important that the nurse introduces the concept of team working early on in the relationship and makes every effort to ensure the patient feels secure with all members of the team.

Similarly, this is an issue when services are not provided outside normal working hours. Nurses must ensure that arrangements are in place for continuing support. Patients and families need to know who to contact and how and what each service contributes to their care.

The third component is breaking the connection. Davies and Oberle (1990) indicate that this most often will be at the point of death. In palliative care, nurses continue to support the family into their bereavement.

In many areas throughout the UK, palliative care is now provided by a combination of service sectors. Connections will be broken as patients are discharged from one aspect of the service to another. Nurse specialists may only be involved in short contacts; they will be discharging many patients before death. Patients and families may feel abandoned if measures to ensure ongoing and seamless support are not in place. It is important that clear arrangements are made with them to ensure that confidence with all service providers is maintained. Equally, patients and families must be reassured that they can contact the nurse again in the future should they need or wish to. By providing their contact details, the nurse ensures that the offer of reconnecting is always available.

Empowerment

Getting to know the patient equips nurses with the knowledge required to assess the patient's current ability or capacity to participate or make choices in their care. This includes ascertaining the patient's attitude towards decision making in relation to their health, the amount of control they prefer in making decisions, their previous experiences, their coping styles and their personal limitations at this time.

Involving patients in their care is fundamental in palliative care and is linked to enhancement of human dignity, increased patient satisfaction, a greater efficacy of health education and improved compliance (Bottorff et al. 2000).

Recognizing this, the code of professional conduct (Nursing and Midwifery Council 2002) now explicitly states 'you must recognise and respect the role of patients and clients as partners in their care and the contribution they can make to it. This involves identifying their preferences regarding care and respecting these within the limits of professional practice, existing legislation, resources and the goals of the therapeutic relationship.'

For patients and families to be offered opportunities and enabled to participate in care, nurses must have the ability, willingness and resources to fully support their involvement. This requires the following.

Knowledge

To provide appropriate suggestions and choices, nurses need to know about the impact of the illness and disease, progression, treatment and prognosis. As an absolute minimum nurses should have a sound knowledge of the core principles of palliative care and know how to access specialist advice. Nurses working in palliative care settings and at specialist levels should possess the knowledge, skills and competencies appropriate to their position as described by Webber (1993).

Effective communication

Skill is essential if patients and families are to be encouraged to discuss sensitive topics and be heard. Patients describe good communicators as those who listen to their particular concerns, who use simple questions that are not too direct, who use open questions and avoid any leading questions and most importantly maintain good eye contact (Bailey and Wilkinson 1998). For this to happen nurses will need to overcome the many barriers to effective communication such as lack of time, knowledge and communication skills training; anxiety about upsetting the patient or not coping; and their own fears of death and dying. Courses and training are clearly valuable, but if used alone will not improve communication. Wilkinson (1999) indicates that all nurses can develop and improve skills if they take every opportunity to develop self-awareness and increase their practice.

Environment

Nurses need to feel supported if they are to engage actively in patient involvement. They require recognition and valuing of patient-focused activities from management, active involvement and role modelling from senior nurses, organization of care to support close patient contact and interdisciplinary collaboration.

Resources

Time, skill mix, equipment and specialist advice can seriously impact on meeting patient choice. For example, the patient may wish to be cared for and die in their own home. In many areas, there is a distinct lack of nursing resources to support this. For others, poor symptom control may prevent a home death.

Attitude

If patients and families are able and wish to participate in care, they must receive the appropriate resources to feel secure and in control. The degree to which the nurse perceives this as a threat or reduction of their power and control may influence their willingness to support their involvement.

In her book, *From novice to expert*, Benner (1984) suggests that expert nurses use their power to empower not to dominate, coerce or control patients. She identifies six different qualities.

Transformative power

The nurse enables patients to see that they have choices and can have control.

Integrative caring

The nurse assists patients to maximize their potential and continue with a meaningful life despite limitations.

Advocacy or enabling

The nurse speaks out on behalf of and with the agreement of the patient.

Healing power

By establishing a healing relationship the nurse mobilizes hope, gains understanding and assists patients and their families to use social, emotional and spiritual support.

Participative/affirmative power

The nurse provides comfort and presence.

Problem solving

By developing a caring relationship the nurse is able to administer creative solutions.

Nurses may not always be aware that their actions reinforce the imbalance of power, for example, asking the patient's preferred name indicates value and respect in the relationship. Yet, many nurses continue to call the patient 'love', 'dear' or 'sweetheart'. In transactional analysis, use of such terms (without the patient's request) by the nurse implies a mothering role. The nurse becomes the mother (adult) speaking to the child (patient) further perpetuating the nurse's position of power (Berne 1964). Nurses indicate that they use such terms as a 'term of endearment' or 'local greeting' and are genuinely unaware of the effect this can have on their relationship. In the author's own service staff ensure that all colleagues are aware of preferred names by using the patient's notes, notice-boards and by mentioning it at every handover.

In support of Benner (1984), Davies and Oberle (1990) indicate that palliative care nurses empower patients and their families through a process of facilitating, encouraging, defusing, mending and giving information.

They work with patients and families facilitating the identification of their own inner resources and individual family strengths. This is an assessment process. The nurse establishes the type and level of involvement that the patient and each family member would like and suggests how they can remain involved and when they may be feeling that they are not able to contribute anything of value. For example, some family members feel unable to participate in the physical aspects of care, indeed it may be inappropriate. The nurse can suggest other ways to help, such as providing social stimulation for the patient through talking, reading, playing games, assisting with hobbies or accompanying on excursions. Alternatively, practical help such as cooking, cleaning, helping with travel arrangements or collecting shopping is equally helpful at this time.

The nurse encourages patients to make decisions or choices about the way in which they want to manage their situation, providing resources and opportunities for them to be involved. For example, if the patient is on an in-patient unit, asking them what visiting arrangements they would like staff to support enables them to control their rest times. An open visiting policy may be welcomed, but for some it places pressure on the family to maintain a presence and can be exhausting for all concerned.

Palliative care nurses attend to the patient's and family's sense of being out of control by recognizing that they are in a situation in which they have had no prior experience and are automatically disadvantaged. Furthermore, in unfamiliar surroundings any sense of control they did have will be further threatened. Nurses reduce this threat if they familiarize the patient and family with their surroundings (if this is not their home) and continue to support their normal home and family life as much as possible.

Patients and families may not have the knowledge necessary to make decisions or understand that they can be involved in care. Although they have access to a much wider range of information than ever before, not all will be accurate or appropriate to that individual. Nurses hand back control to the patient and their family by accessing and providing the information they require for decision making and participating in care. This may include information that is traditionally within the medical domain such as information relating to diagnosis, treatment, disease progression or prognosis. In palliative care, nurses are encouraged to discuss such issues and the emphasis is on open communication. However, it should be recognized that there are some settings where medical dominance prevails and nurses may not be 'allowed' to engage in such discussions. Wherever possible nurses should work collaboratively with their medical colleagues, but not collude in any avoidance of patients' enquiries. Nurses are personally accountable to the patient and have a duty to provide truthful information about their condition (United Kingdom Central Council 1996).

Patients should be fully involved with decision making and in their own care. The possibilities are vast, ranging from contributing to assessment and care planning to undertaking self-care activities such as self-medication (Bird and Hassall 1993). One example that illustrates the former and demonstrates how care can be substantially improved is documented by

Cadd *et al.* (2000). In their study of bowel management on a palliative in-patient unit, they showed that patient preferences were rarely incorporated in care plans. They imply that if nurses improved their techniques for eliciting and documenting this information, the use of medications and invasive procedures might be reduced.

Some self-care activities require learning new skills or different ways of doing things. Nurses can help patients and families by working alongside them, for example, teaching and supervising until they have gained the confidence to be independent.

At times, patients and families may be extremely upset, confused or angry. Nurses will be required to defuse situations by giving permission to express negative reactions. These feelings may sometimes be projected towards the nurse. Nurses who understand how patients and families may react when under stress, who have developed their skills of communicating in difficult situations and who receive appropriate support, will be able to respond sensitively rather than defensively; the nurse–patient relationship will remain intact (Benner and Wrubel 1989).

At times conflicts arise within the family when reactions of individual members appear to be at odds with each other. By working closely with the family, facilitating discussion, helping them to understand why and how each are reacting and how they can overcome such rifts, nurses empower the whole family to remain united as a team. Davies and Oberle (1990) refer to this as mending.

Finding meaning

As patients and their families begin to acknowledge the inevitability of death, they may start to question the spiritual aspects of their life such as the meaning of the illness, their life and their death. It is common for the patient to want to consider what they have or have not achieved throughout their life.

This can be extremely distressing as they focus on the aspects of their life such as regrets, missed opportunities and unrealized dreams. They may consider their future to be one of only illness, suffering and loss and may have great difficulty in continuing to invest in a life worth living. On the other hand, it can be a time for growth, hopes and fulfilling wishes and can be a life-enhancing experience as patients and families recognize, value and attend to the more important aspects of their life.

Nurses can help patients and their families to find meaning by acknow-ledging death and focusing on living (Davies and Oberle 1990).

However, nurses often do not know how to help or choose to ignore the issue (Heaven and Maguire 1997; Cobb 2001). Reasons include

- poor awareness of spirituality and the signs of spiritual distress;
- fear of incompetence;
- lack of resources, such as access to a chaplain or religious representative;
- lack of time, low priority;
- inadequate communication skills;
- a focus on the physical aspects of care;
- the nursing process and documentation of care;
- environment.

In a study by Heaven and Maguire (1997), patients in a hospice were found to be less willing to disclose psychological, social and spiritual concerns than their physical concerns to nurses and furthermore sometimes deliberately withheld such information. Inadequate communication skills of nurses led to presumptions about patients' needs and difficulties in recognizing and documenting spiritual concerns. Heaven and Maguire (1997) suggest that non-disclosure may have been a consequence of the hospice emphasis on symptom control through which patients learn that professionals are not interested in other issues. Additionally, patients may not wish to overburden vulnerable staff. They concluded by saying that non-disclosure should not be interpreted as a lack of distress for many of the most anxious and depressed patients were amongst those who withheld their concerns.

Developing self-awareness of what spirituality can mean to others and what it means to them enables nurses to recognize spiritual needs. Developing effective communication skills will enable nurses to ascertain and attend to needs. Nurses should be prepared to enter into dialogue about such sensitive issues and be willing to engage at an emotional level. However, they must be supported appropriately to enable them to have time to listen and the courage to be alongside someone in their suffering.

Nurses must be alert for signs of spiritual distress such as anger, anxiety, guilt, loss, despair, isolation and alienation. At times it may present as a physical symptom, such as uncontrolled pain, as the following case illustrates.

John, aged 91, was referred to the palliative care nurse from the care of the elderly unit for assessment of his pain. He had been diagnosed as having inoperable lung cancer 2 months before the referral. Despite trials of steroids, anti-inflammatory drugs and escalating doses of opiates, he continued to report severe pain. He had become tearful, but was refusing to talk to staff.

On examining the notes before her visit, the nurse noted that he had changed his religion within the last 3 weeks. At first, John refused to speak to the nurse; he turned his body away from her and closed his eyes. The nurse asked if it might be all right if she stayed with him for a while. No reply. After 20 minutes, John opened his eyes. He asked the nurse if she was religious, as she was wearing a crucifix. John told her that he had found no support in religion. He became anxious and close to tears. The nurse encouraged him to go on. He explained how his mother had conceived him after being raped by her brother. Most of his childhood had been spent being told that he was the devil's spawn and now he was frightened of 'meeting his maker'. He had not told anyone and was scared to discuss this with the priest who had baptized him. The nurse was able to arrange and be present during a meeting with the priest. Over the next 3 weeks, John's pain gradually decreased to the level where he required regular weak opiates. John and the priest continued to meet regularly until his death.

For many patients and families religion is a source of great comfort. Enabling them to continue to practise their beliefs will be essential for their spiritual health and well-being. Nurses can facilitate this by clearly identifying patients' and families' religious beliefs and establishing how they personally choose to practise and how they wish to continue in this particular setting. Accessing a chaplain for further support may be required. Assumptions based on religious affiliation should be avoided at all costs.

For others, religion may be the source of their distress. They may be experiencing a crisis of faith or like John be fearful of punishment for past behaviours. Nurses can help patients by assisting them to identify the source of their distress and where appropriate helping them to access support from a chaplain or other member of the religious community if appropriate.

As patients and families acknowledge a limited prognosis, time becomes more precious and anything that wastes time can cause further distress. Nurses can help patients and families to use the time they have left by focusing on living. By helping patients to identify what is most important to them, nurses can assist in fulfilling realistic hopes and dreams. Sensitive planning and prioritizing of activities will enable more time to be spent on the activities that are most important to the patient and their family at this time.

Doing for

Although promoting self-care has been the main feature of this chapter, there will be times when the patient and family are no longer able to continue unaided and the nurse will need to take charge of certain aspects or of all care the patient requires. Most often this relates to the physical aspects of care such as pain and symptom control or enhancing patient comfort through physical nursing care. For some patients it will involve planning and co-ordinating packages of care. In this aspect of their role, the nurse uses all their professional knowledge and skills in delivering care that promotes patient and family comfort and enhances quality of life. Most commonly, but not exclusively, it is associated with end-of-life care. Most patients and families want to continue caring themselves for as long as possible, although some may be relieved that someone else will take on the responsibility. It should come as no surprise that many patients and families are reluctant to hand over this aspect of care. Nurses can ease this transition by continuously demonstrating that the care they plan and deliver remains focused on the individual patient and their family and that their participation in care is encouraged.

Most nursing care in the UK is process based. Patient care is assessed, planned and evaluated. Wherever possible this should be in partnership with the patient. If the patient is unable to contribute because of confusion or unconsciousness, it will be important that the family are included in discussions relating to care planning. The nurse's prior knowledge of the patient and their relationship with the family will be essential in this respect.

Taking time to explain, providing information and offering suggestions and choices remain key components at this time. One must stress that for many patients decision making might be too tiring and they may not want the burden of the responsibility. For others, as long as they can communicate they may still wish to continue despite being bed-bound and dependent on nurses for all their care. Nurses can continue to offer choices even if only about how the patient would like to spend their day or how they would like to attend to their personal hygiene needs.

Family members often feel quite anxious at this time, wanting to participate in care but not quite knowing how. They often remark that they are worried that they will hurt the patient. Nurses can continue to involve them by creating opportunities for them to work alongside her in activities such as bed bathing and re-positioning the patient. The nurse can teach them activities that they may wish to continue such as gentle massage, skin, nail and oral care and assisting the patient to eat or drink or if this is no longer possible they can be shown how to keep the mouth moist and clean.

Preserving own integrity

Providing patient-focused care for palliative and terminally ill patients and their families is challenging. It exposes nurses to great distress and intense emotional situations. They face situations that may remind them of personal experiences, their own family members or of their own mortality.

For nurses to remain effective and to have the courage to be alongside someone in their suffering, they need to feel confident that what they do is helping to make a difference. Without it they are at great risk of stress and burnout (Vachon 1987). It is their confidence that enables nurses to be open and compassionate towards patients and families, further increasing their effectiveness. Nurses develop confidence by maintaining feelings of self-worth and self-esteem and energy levels. Davies and Oberle (1990) indicate that this is achieved by looking inward, valuing self and acknowledging own reactions.

Self-awareness is essential for nurses in palliative care; it enables them to understand and recognize their feelings, behaviours and reactions and how these might influence care. Nurses who have not developed this or do not work in settings that promote opportunities to reflect may encounter great personal distress or may avoid difficult situations, escalating their feelings of inadequacy. By periodically looking inward nurses are able to reflect on their own thoughts and beliefs about the meaning of life, suffering and death and how it relates to the work that they do.

By valuing self, nurses recognize that what they do is making a difference. They might receive confirmation in the form of a smile, verbal feedback from the patient or family or praise from colleagues. It is important that senior nurses facilitate this by ensuring work is organized in a way that promotes close patient contact, highlighting feedback such as thank you letters and providing regular formal feedback. In some settings, debriefing sessions at the end of each shift provide the forum to review and value each other's input.

Valuing self also requires that nurses pay attention to life outside of the workplace and maintain a balance between work with home, family and social activities (Vachon 1987).

Nurses need to be satisfied that they have done the right thing for the right reasons. This requires the ability to continually assess and acknowledge thoughts, feelings, actions and reactions. In addition to reflecting on their personal feelings, it enables nurses to review the quality of care and identify areas for personal and professional development. Reflecting at this level often requires facilitating. The benefits of clinical supervision are well documented (Teasdale and Brocklehurst 2001). However, in many settings nurses do not have access to an appropriately trained supervisor. Other support such as debriefing, case reviews, reflective diaries and staff-support sessions, whilst not an alternative to clinical supervision, may be helpful.

Conclusion

Regardless of the setting, all nurses can provide effective palliative nursing. By getting to know the patient and family, establishing a relationship based on trust and providing opportunities for their involvement, nurses can help them to feel valued and in control in an otherwise unfamiliar and unpredictable situation. Working alongside patients and their families, assisting them to meet their specific needs and achieve their goals, is the very essence and reward of palliative nursing.

References

Bailey K and Wilkinson S (1998). Cancer patients perceptions of nurses' communication skills. *International Journal of Palliative Nursing* 4: 300–5.

Benner P (1984). *From Novice to Expert.* Addison-Wesley, California.

Benner P and Wrubel J (1989). *The Primacy of Caring.* Addison-Wesley, California.

Berne E (1964). *Games People Play.* Penguin Books, Middlesex.

Bird C and Hassall J (1993). *Self Administration of Drugs.* Scutari Press, London.

Bottorff J, Steele R, Davies B, Porterfield P, Garossino C and Shaw M (2000). Facilitating day to day decision-making in palliative care. *Cancer Nursing* 23: 141–50.

Cadd A, Keatinge D, Henssen M, O'Brien L, Parkes D, Rohr Y (2000). Assessment and documentation of bowel management in palliative care incorporating patient preferences into the care regimen. *Journal of Clinical Nursing* 9: 228–335.

Cobb M (2001). *The dying soul, spiritual care at the end of life.* Open University Press, Buckingham.

Davies B and Oberle K (1990). Dimensions of the supportive role of the nurse in palliative care. *Oncology Nurse Forum* 1: 87–94.

Dingman SK, Williams M, Fosbinder D and Warnick M (1999). Implementing a caring model to improve patient satisfaction. *Journal of Nursing Administration* 29: 30–7.

Ellis S (1999). The patient centred care model: holistic/multiprofessional/reflective. *British Journal of Nursing* 8: 296–301.

Heaven C and Maguire P (1997). Disclosure of concerns by hospice patients and their identification by nurses. *Palliative Medicine* 11: 283–90.

Lugton J and Kindlen M (1999). *Palliative Care, The Nursing Role.* Churchill Livingstone, Edinburgh.

Morse J (1991). Negotiating commitment and involvement in the nurse–patient relationship. *Journal of Advanced Nursing* 16: 455–68.

Nursing and Midwifery Council (2002). *Code of Professional Conduct.*

Teasdale K and Brocklehurst N (2001). Clinical supervision and support for nurses: an evaluation study. *Journal of Advanced Nursing* **33**: 216–24.

United Kingdom Central Council (1996). *Guidelines for Professional Practice.*

Vachon M (1987). *Occupational Stress in the Care of the Critically Ill, the Dying, and the Bereaved.* Hemisphere Publishing Corporation, USA.

Webber J (1993). The evolving role of the Macmillan nurse. Unpublished paper, Cancer Relief, Macmillan Fund.

Wilkinson S (1999). Scering Plough clinical lecture communication: it makes a difference. *Cancer Nursing* **22**: 17–20.

11

Palliative care social work

Lindsey Napier

Introduction

Social work in palliative care sets out to understand and respond to the social dimensions of the experience of people with life-threatening illness. Three basic aims are

- to address the social concerns and problems of seriously ill and dying people and their families;
- to create and strengthen the social supportiveness of their environment;
- to find ways of redressing the social inequalities that permeate the experience of illness and dying.

The ways in which social workers fulfil these aims are shaped by the populations they serve, their country and place of work, diverse cultural values, the people with whom they work as colleagues, the requirements and provisions of social policies and the scope for discretion in how they work. Much of the work is conducted in alliance and partnership with others. Much is conducted in negotiation.

Social work has to reckon with its local histories and with how it is currently perceived. Its histories are bound up with the wish to do good—for example, to redress social inequalities, to enhance people's quality of life, to stop violence or to provide social resources for health and wellbeing. Social work is also bound up with the fact that it is not 'innocent', that it is part of controlling regimes of governance. The idea of meeting a 'social worker' is not always greeted positively. It often conjures up pictures of 'removals'—removal of old people to nursing homes, removal of children damaged by abuse and neglect to foster care. It also conjures up pictures of alleged failure to remove—adults because they present a public health or mental health hazard, infants and children because allegedly too little was done too late. Apprehension, shame, anger, resignation and sadness abound.

Social work is accustomed to playing this conflictual or 'eccentric' role as Oliviere (2001) has called it. Over all the years of hospice and palliative care development, social work has examined its will and capacity to 'put the client first', for example, in terms of its responsiveness to racial and cultural diversity. Approaches to practice have been developed that demand attention to the processes of discrimination and exclusion—on the grounds of age, class, sexuality, race and gender, for example—and to the aims and processes of empowerment. Social work has also become circumspect of the comfortable certainties and expert power that modernist approaches promise and has developed approaches that prize uncertainty, curiosity, diversity and provisional knowledge. These have immediate resonance for work with ill and dying people, where uncertainty abounds and there is still much silencing. Sharing fears and hopes as people live towards death is still difficult. These approaches challenge fixed ideas about who are the primary experts on dying and death (Napier 2000).

The policy context

In a market place of care, where people are positioned as consumers and users, and social workers in many settings have become 'gate-keeping enablers' (see Harris and McDonald 2000 for a comparison of Australia and the UK, for example) social work has to give substance to the words choice, control, participation and empowerment in ways that also address diversity, disadvantage and discrimination.

The reality is that people who use palliative care resources are not 'sovereign consumers', able to pick and choose freely in the market place or able to switch from one service to another and take their business elsewhere. At times of critical illness, it is likely that people do need experts to know what is wrong and to advise what may help. Trust must often be conceded. The presence of trust may be an important part of the relationship between provider and user. The presence of trust can simplify complexity and reduce apprehension, doubt and fear.

While consumers have responsibilities as well as rights, the reality is that choice is often non-existent or severely constrained. While what may be wanted by a family for the last days of their relative's life is a place of quietness and privacy, the noisy thoroughfare of a shared hospital ward may be all that is available. As well, there is often conflict over whose choice is 'the right choice' (Small and Rhodes 2000), for choices and decisions are commonly made within relationships. For example, some members of a family may be at odds with others and with 'the professionals' in their interpretation of what their ill relative wishes but cannot communicate. They may consider referral of their relative to palliative care as nothing short of abandonment and press for the continuation of invasive treatment.

Again, people are differently socially situated, with differing perceptions about their rights and entitlements. For social work, there is a persuasive view that 'all who need should receive' regardless of their purchasing power, or their confidence to exert personal authority in professional encounters.

It may be helpful, following Saltman (1994), to distinguish between a commercial approach to care provision, in which consumers exercise *choice* in a market-driven system and a political approach, in which users are given a *voice* in a system, which ensures their participation and empowerment. Empowerment, however defined, implies an active process, and is evident in models of care that emphasize 'the interdependent status of service users as citizens requiring assistance but with the right to autonomous decision-making' (Barnes and Walker 1996). User empowerment can aim to

- empower people at an individual level—to redress the balance of power between patient and professional and to enable people to have a greater say in their own treatment and care;

- empower people at a collective level—to increase the participation of users of services in decisions about their design, management and review, or as citizens, in wider consultation about services and priorities (Small and Rhodes 2000).

I shall examine social work practice with respect to both these levels of engagement with people with life-threatening illness and progressive disorders. It is worth noting that often people do not have a free choice about how they are addressed—as clients, patients, consumers, users or as fellow human beings. Here I shall call them people who are ill, people with progressive disease, people who are perhaps dying, either alone or in the company of people to whom they matter.

I select fragments of social work practice—from the work of personal assistance, of creating supportive environments and of building social resources for wellbeing at the end of life—to provide pictures of the social dimensions of ill people's experience and of the breadth of a social work response.

Personal assistance

Personal assistance forms a significant part of social work in palliative care. Empowerment approaches in social work start from the assumption that people have potential strengths to call on when illness strikes and death is not far away. This does not diminish the requirement for social work to offer personal assistance. Such assistance aims to ensure that predictable and reliable personal, social and material support are in place; to help people who speak different languages or 'languages' of custom, ritual and meaning to communicate more clearly with one another; to work within and often beyond the social rules to help a person who is dying try and realize their final dreams and visions; to recognize and offer skilled assistance so that a family can if they wish confront family conflicts 'before it is too late'; to help people find paths towards reconciliation or sometimes separation; and to negotiate on people's behalf with social institutions like workplaces, schools and government departments, for example, for understanding, 'days off' or safer, health-giving housing.

Social work places ideas about crisis, loss, grief and bereavement within an appreciation of people's diverse and unequal social circumstances. As for all who work in palliative care, however, all the understanding in the world is of limited value unless we are able to start where people 'are at' and to 'connect' with the person dying and with the people surrounding them. The road being travelled after all is altogether unfamiliar and for the person dying, the final stage has to be travelled alone. It is all too easy to stand in people's way and like others, social workers are only effective when we facilitate and do not impede. This includes being open to talk appropriately about dying and death.

To illustrate social work in practice, I select the apparently simple task of assisting people gain understanding of their situation through the processes of offering and requesting information and of questioning.

Offering information

Understanding can help give a sense of control and can offer the chance for a person to make choices and plans. The opportunity to understand depends in part on the opening of doors to information. While social workers are likely to assume that most people want information about their condition and the resources available to support them, they know that there are times when the responsibility of possessing information is too burdensome. The only way some people can contemplate a distressing and uncertain future may be by putting all their trust and decisions in others' hands.

People come with differing prior experience of asking questions and seeking information. One person may never have felt entitled to ask questions. When they did, and spoke up, their reward may have been severe punishment. Another may have always set the agenda, decided both on the questions and the correct answers. Finding themselves ignorant and lost may be bewildering and anger making. Others may be required to defer to those 'in authority' to ask the questions: choice may not be free but bound by particular family rules or group custom. Yet again, the experience of being given information may not always have been an invitation to understanding. Rather, it may have been a way of being dismissed—'Take this and go!'—so as not to waste the precious time of officials.

Providing information is not a neutral process. The practitioner makes decisions about to whom they offer information and about which information is offered and which withheld. Who, for example, is best placed to share information about a parent's imminent death with a child? In a review of her work with a group of 40 families immediately before, during and immediately after the death of a parent, Lee (2000) concluded that wherever possible the information is best given to children 'by the parent who loves and cares for them, otherwise by someone else whom the child knows and trusts. The information needs to come from someone who has credibility for the child.'

Information giving is as much a process as an event.

Requesting information

In the process of conducting social assessment, social workers make many requests for information. For assessment to be empowering, social workers aim for it to be transparent and mutual. They must be explicit about purpose. First of all, there is an effort to be alert to people's prior experience of 'being questioned'. Some people know that the motives for asking questions are not always benign: they may recall awful consequences to being questioned. Resistance to being asked more questions may conceal a person's deep frustration at being asked repeatedly for the same information (Sanderson 1998). Lunn and Feldon (1998), discussing the work of a palliative care unit for people with AIDS, report on the value of initial assessment being carried out by the ill person themselves. This may in any case produce greater benefit by way of take up of services when they are offered some control over which professionals they wish to seek out.

In a different setting, that may not be possible. Southern (1998), for example, identifies how, regardless of need, withdrawal into oneself may be the only way available to a person to manage the overwhelming experience of an unfamiliar large hospital, long journeys to reach it, demanding treatment schedules, frequent changes of staff and having to cope alone. Providing a safe environment, a regular place to talk and some continuity of personnel may be the minimal prerequisites to removing barriers of suspicion enough for the ill person to let someone 'in'.

Supporting critical questioning

In the course of their work with a person who is dying, it may be appropriate for the social worker to support a person 'critically question' the sources of the beliefs and feelings that are weighing them down—for example, a person may believe that staying positive is essential for their very survival. They may be afraid of 'giving' cancer to others. They may feel themselves to be a constant burden regardless of objective evidence or feel bound to keep going regardless of their own private wishes. It may be possible for the social worker to encourage examination of the social sources of such beliefs and feelings and for the person to consider whether at this point in their lives they need be bound by them.

Croft (2000) has reported that the main concern for most of the more than a hundred women with whom she worked as they approached death was their internalization of responsibility and concern for others. This was so regardless of age. In her experience, ' … the decisions that most women make around their illness, treatment and impending death, relate to how these are going to affect others and not primarily themselves'. Croft considered that while this can be positive for women, it also raises dilemmas about whether it is possible to provide support for them to give some priority to themselves.

In presenting her data, Croft observed that she was not intending to generalize about all women or to exclude men. She alerts the practitioner to the diversity of human experience. Practitioners note that some widowers, in their dying, are pained for the fact that soon they will no longer be able to protect their children from mortality. Young men may have to struggle with feelings that by dying, they are betraying their young families, because they believe that their role is to provide and protect. It may be helpful for the practitioner to listen out for the burden being carried by the weight of these social scripts.

Creating and strengthening supportive environments

Offering social support

Social work is usually involved in assessing the adequacy of social support for the ill person and their family. On first consideration, this may seem like a routine task of seeking out information, making referral, determining eligibility, linking, advocating, negotiating and working within and beyond the bounds of limited resources to provide a 'package of support'. What are the social dimensions of social support? One definition might be that social support is about relationships and what they offer, in terms of practical, emotional and informational assistance and in terms of when such assistance is offered. Is support continuous or only when there is distress? Social workers are wary both of shared meanings and of shared understanding as to who should and can provide what. The reasons people have for providing social support vary enormously—love, altruism, obligation, guilt, tradition or position in a hierarchy, for example. Working to understand the social rules that underpin the offering and receiving of support in a person's cultural community is important. For example, if reciprocity has always been expected in a person's family relationships, they may turn in increasing frailty to formal services rather than feel they are violating accepted custom.

As a social worker I do not assume that support from the 'informal sphere' is automatically possible, even when policy may require this. People may not command the necessary social resources—networks and connections, knowledge and understanding, freedom to be absent from paid employment, money for airfares or time—especially over a long period. Sometimes the will to provide support is not there: home may have been a place of violence or neglect. Support, however generously offered, is not always a 'good thing'. For all sorts of reasons, people can make a painful situation worse—resolute cheerfulness, for example, is not always supportive.

Added to that, for people to be treated with respect, as active subjects, social workers resist the idea that social support is something to be applied (a bit like a poultice) to people whose situation is deficient in some way and who passively wait for formal services to plug the gaps. The assumption that support is unidirectional is of course true at particular times of critical illness and difficulty. However support takes different forms. For example, it is well known that old people who are parents and guardians continue to support their 'children' through money, property, company for grandchildren, interest—and often affection! They are frequently the net givers over time in families. Support may still be reciprocal, just differing in nature. The danger of failing to recognize this is to negate the still active contribution people who are very ill may be making to their relationships.

Again, in collaboration with colleagues, attention must be paid to the relative inclusiveness and social supportiveness of the environment where formal care and treatment are provided—the environment of hospital waiting rooms, patient transport services or day units, for example. This leads to social work's involvement in the policy dimensions of social support: just as health and illness are unequally distributed, so too are the social resources with which to support ill people and their families. Saunders' concept of 'total pain' recognized that to be effective social support must take account of people's varying social circumstances. Palliative care may be the final opportunity to redistribute social support, of whatever sort.

Supporting collective self-help

For some people who find themselves in 'the same boat' the benefits of meeting together are well known. The impetus to start a group often springs from a wish by a few determined people to prevent others experiencing the isolation and loneliness they have felt. It may simply be that even though professionals try their best, they cannot understand the personal experience. Only those 'going through it' can. This is what Gray *et al.* (1997) called 'instant bonding', 'a kind of connecting that did not require words'. Fear of having to cope alone after multiple losses of friends was considered by Fulton *et al.* (1996) to have been a significant motivation for group participation by Australian men living with AIDS. Identifying with each other's condition and experience may lead to an emergent solidarity that can assist group members resist stigma.

To be helpful, the nature of reciprocal support must be specific. In discussion of self-help groups of women with breast cancer, for example, Gray *et al.* (1997) observed that deaths of members proved the hardest challenge. The capacity of groups to incorporate loss and death more explicitly into group life was tenuous. The groups described by McLeod (1999) were established specifically for women with secondary breast cancer. In these groups, where deaths of group members are part of the life of groups, talk of dying is as normal as talk of treatment experience and hopes for recovery. 'Experienced empathy' is possible.

Social workers often assist at the formative stage of self-help groups. They may judge that there are particular benefits for members when groups are facilitated. Kraus (1998) explains that, when group membership continually changed, her presence as a facilitator provided a sense of safety and continuity, together with a sense of security and freedom for members to express feelings, including about the news of the death of a member. The group provided a place for remembrance and the assurance that surviving members would be remembered when they died.

Kraus's observation that group members themselves became both expert and therapist is reinforced by Firth (1998), who reports on facilitated group work with young people. She points out that groups are a 'natural environment' for young people. 'Young people like to help one another and peer affirmation is much more powerful than adult reinforcement.'

Self-help initiatives can raise the status of experiential knowledge (McLeod 1999). People's sources of knowledge and power come from within.

Working with families

A key component of social work in palliative care is with the people who matter most to the ill or dying person (Sheldon 2000). For many the term 'family' best describes these people. For others the term 'family' is conflictual, empty of meaning or excluding of the person or people that most matter. 'The ties that bind' may or may not be those of blood or legal contract. Respecting diversity requires social workers to work with whoever is important and to restrain any tendency to convey normative perceptions of who belongs in a family and set normative expectations of its members.

In palliative care families are acknowledged both as the primary providers of care of their ill relative, and with them, as the 'unit of care' (World Health Organization 1990). They are entitled to ask for care, both to enable them to continue providing care and to assist them cope throughout the illness and achieve wellbeing in bereavement. The terms on which such care is based is often called partnership. Thus the ways in which social work relates to families must acknowledge this interdependence.

In some social policy debates, there has been a tendency to influence people to think of care as a 'burden', where dependency has been constructed as undesirable. It is true that there are costs to caring—to health, income and life choices. Yet this label of 'burden' may not describe the experience accurately: the relationships between cared for and carers may be the key to the wellbeing of *both* parties.

For social workers there must be wariness of labelling families in ways that question their 'normality' or oversimplify the relations of care. Approaches that assume potential underlying 'psychosocial morbidity', that differentiate 'functional' from 'dysfunctional' families and assume professional authority to improve 'family functioning' are justifiable only if the labels are found to be helpful by the ill or dying person and the people who matter to them. Similarly, there must be a rejection of too readily labelling families as 'compliant' or 'non-compliant', when that may reveal that they have not been involved in determining the terms of the partnership. This is especially so if families are attempting to manage when stretched because of constraints in other parts of their lives—employment demands, poor public transport, competing caring responsibilities or little money, for example.

In writing of their work with families, social workers have pointed out that the aim of assisting family members to communicate more freely is to release their existing strengths. Over weeks and months of necessary surrender to a passivity of 'active treatment', the ill person and their family may have lost touch with their normal confidence to take control and act on their own behalf (Monroe 1998). During the final phase of the person's illness, people close to the dying person may have to cope with unpredictable and rapidly changing expectations of the likely path of illness, including where the final hours or days of life may take place (Clark and Cooper 2000). All their energy may have been consumed by trying to 'fit in with the system', a system that may be unable or unwilling to cater for diverse cultural needs. For the family's confidence to be restored and their strength to be galvanized, the social worker may be most helpful by being informer, coach, advocate and a reliable, safe person to steer them through the maze.

Systems approaches to family work aim to develop capacity to cope. In strengths approaches, the focus is on identifying what people have done and can do in order to survive, contain and change (Saleebey 1997, 2001). Thinking about families from an assumption of strengths and resilience is not to ignore or minimize problems. The strict expectation however is to avoid labelling the person and those who matter into categories of illness or deficit; rather the expectation is to acknowledge the resilience of people, their ability to endure and survive in the face of adversity. This is difficult to accomplish. The evidence for the effectiveness of such approaches in palliative care social work is yet to be documented. To some, it may seem at best alarmingly naïve and at worst to risk denying issues of inequality and conflict. It does however lend respect to the idea of partnership.

Building social resources for wellbeing at the end of life

Dying is a universal human experience. Learning about living and dying and discovering the multiple meanings that people make of them seems a sensible activity. How can this happen? What social and cultural changes are needed so that knowledge about life and living, death and dying, which everyone has to accomplish, is 'part of the community'?

There are many 'communities of knowledge' and interest groups in the life situation of people who are dying—people who are approaching the end of their lives, their friends and families, hospice volunteers, clergy, palliative care teams, self-help organizations and professional groups. The most important teachers of a 'dialogue on living and dying' may be dying people themselves.

The evidence from community development work is that cultural change sometimes starts with just one pebble being thrown into the pond. Social work has a long community work tradition, including in community and public health. Such work links personal assistance and personal troubles with public issues. It aims for people to gain greater control over their lives; to support people in *their* identified struggles and to stand alongside them; to give priority to the most disadvantaged; and to intervene early in order to stop individual problems and individualistic responses developing (Jackson *et al.* 1989).

Achieving participation in dialogue is not easy: language, racism, shyness, lack of knowledge and experience and fear of democracy, for example, can make for difficulty. It requires extensive groundwork, not least to build trust. It requires information that can be used. Listening to and understanding the diversity of needs, issues and aspirations identified before taking action on a few common issues is crucial to enhance participation. Establishing sustained individual relationships are the basis for the worker engaging as a non-directive facilitator. Having fun, not surprisingly, is an essential part of working together (Lane 1990).

Broader community work in palliative care could aim to accomplish, say—a better understanding of the diverse customs and values that people of different faiths and cultures hold about dying; a recognition of the collective losses suffered by families, groups and communities from different countries and cultures and ways found helpful for remembering them; the creation of a common stock of knowledge about the processes of dying and death; and a demand for greater attention in health and social policy to the social rights and needs of people at the end of their lives. Such dialogue would also, most likely, create expectations that services become more adequate and more responsive to diverse need.

Reflection

This raises questions of values—'We need to change the assumption that dying people are no longer of any economic value and therefore of no value at all', commented a group of social workers recently. It poses issues for social policy—empowerment is not an alternative to adequate resourcing of services and does not remove the responsibilities of those who produce them (Barnes and Walker 1996). The question of how social policy should address questions like 'What are we all prepared to pay for everyone at the end of life?' is surely a question for discussion in diverse communities. Creating such a ripple of dialogue may sound fanciful, though why not?

This is how hospices started—small, diverse, local, the work of a committed few.

These are the thoughts of one person, speaking from one place in social work. It is a contribution to a dialogue about 'a voice for the voiceless'.

Acknowledgement

The author acknowledges the comments of the Palliative Care Social Workers Special Interest Group, New South Wales, Australia on this chapter.

References

Barnes M and Walker A (1996). Consumerism versus empowerment: a principled approach to the involvement of older service users. *Policy and Politics*, 24, 375–93.

Clark M and Cooper L (2000). Unexpected changes. *Palliative Care* (Newsletter, Australian Association of Social Workers (NSW)), 2, 20–2.

Croft S (2000). How can I leave them? Towards an empowering social work practice with women who are dying. In Fawcett B, Galloway M and Perrins J (ed.) *Feminism and Social Work in the Year 2000: Conflicts and Controversies*, pp. 74–89. Department of Applied Social Studies, Bradford.

Firth P (1998). A long-term closed group for young people. In Oliviere D, Hargreaves R and Monroe B (ed.) *Good Practices in Palliative Care*, pp. 86–93. Ashgate Arena, Aldershot.

Fulton G, Madden C and Minichiello V (1996). The social construction of anticipatory grief. *Social Science and Medicine*, 43, 1349–58.

Gray R, Fitch M, Davis C and Phillips C (1997). A qualitative study of breast cancer self-help groups. *Psycho-Oncology*, 6, 279–89.

Harris J and McDonald C (2000). Post-Fordism, the Welfare State and the personal social services: A comparison of Australia and Britain. *British Journal of Social Work*, 30, 51–70.

Jackson T, Mitchell S and Wright M (1989). The community development continuum. *Community Health Studies*, XIII, 66–73.

Kellehear A (1999). *Health Promoting Palliative Care*. Oxford University Press, Melbourne.

Kraus F (1998). Ongoing group work for people with terminal illness. In Oliviere D, Hargreaves R and Monroe B (ed.) *Good Practices in Palliative Care*, pp. 76–80. Ashgate Arena, Aldershot.

Lane M (1990). Community work with immigrant groups. *Australian Social Work*, 43, 33–8.

Lee M (2000). What do we say to the children? *Palliative Care* (Newsletter, Australian Association of Social Workers (NSW)), 2, 15–18.

Lunn S and Feldon C (1998). A patient-focused approach to assessment. In Oliviere D, Hargreaves R and Monroe B (ed.) *Good Practices in Palliative Care*, pp. 40–43. Ashgate Arena, Aldershot.

McLeod E (1999). Self help support groups in secondary breast cancer—a new UK initiative. *European Journal of Palliative Care*, 6, 103–5.

McLeod E and Bywaters P (2000). *Social Work, Health and Equality*. Routledge, London.

Monroe B (1998). Social work in palliative care. In Doyle D, Hanks G and MacDonald N (ed.) *Oxford Textbook of Palliative Medicine*, pp. 867–80. Oxford University Press, Oxford.

Napier L (2000). For ever beyond. In Fawcett B, Featherstone B, Fook J and Rossiter A (ed.) *Practice and Research in Social Work. Postmodern Feminist Perspectives*, pp. 159–75. Routledge, London.

Oliviere D (2001). The social worker in palliative care—the 'eccentric' role. *Progress in Palliative Care*, 9, 237–41.

Saleebey D (ed.) (1997). *The Strengths Perspective in Social Work Practice* (2nd edition). Longman, New York.

Saleebey D (2001). Practicing the strengths perspective: everyday tools and resources. *Families in Society*, 82, 221–2.

Saltman R (1994). Patient choice and patient empowerment. *International Journal of Health Services*, 24, 201–29.

Sanderson J (1998). A family-based approach to assessment. In Oliviere D, Hargreaves R and Monroe B (ed.) *Good Practices in Palliative Care*, pp. 33–40. Ashgate Arena, Aldershot.

Sheldon F (2000). Dimensions of the role of the social worker in palliative care. *Palliative Medicine*, 14, 491–8.

Small N and Rhodes P (2000). *Too Ill to Talk? User Involvement and Palliative Care*. Routledge, London.

Southern P (1998). Assessment in a hospital, multi-professional palliative care team. In Oliviere D, Hargreaves R and Monroe B (ed.) *Good Practices in Palliative Care*, pp. 28–33. Ashgate Arena, Aldershot.

World Health Organization (1990). Cancer pain relief and palliative care. Technical Report 804. World Health Organization, Geneva.

12

Palliative care and chaplaincy

Peter W. Speck

Introduction

It is difficult to envisage an effective chaplaincy, or spiritual care, service that does not strive to be truly interactive with the recipients of that care. To provide spiritual care that is relevant, meaningful and supportive to the patient necessitates a process of discernment of what the person's needs might be, exploration of the options appropriate to meeting those needs and then engaging together in the relevant ritual or activity.

The sensitive nature of this interaction becomes even more important when one considers the wide variety of ways in which people will try to make sense of critical events in their lives. Within the context of a crisis, such as the diagnosis of a life-threatening illness, people will usually revert to previous patterns of understanding. They will also have developed some strategies for helping them come through a crisis. If these are of use in the current event, then all well and good. However, if they do not provide what the person needs then they may well seek new or alternative approaches. Within the person's inner life a similar re-examination may be taking place in terms of trying to understand why this event should have happened; does it have any purpose for them and their family and what resources can they draw upon for support and guidance? The impact of the disease and the treatment offered may also add to this experience so that it can feel as if the person's very identity is being threatened or changed.

The inner dialogue that can take place within many patients is a very private and personal affair but the concept of narrative can be useful in understanding this process.

Narrative theory focuses on the valuations that a person identifies as being the key units of meaning in their life and that provide ways for people to make sense of themselves through stories. These stories often run in the individual's own mind as they identify what is important in the process of thinking about their life situation. Hermans (1992) expounds a theoretical understanding of this process when he describes the '*dialogical self*' that is multiple and embedded in dialogue. We tend to take for granted that the self is singular and that, to some extent, *I* create *my* life story. While my life story may have many characters it is a single *I* who creates them. According to Hermans instead of an individual, rational self, the person is endowed with multiple storytelling selves, each in dialogue with the others (Hermans *et al.* 1992). Within the context of a new life experience the individual will review that experience from the perspective of their various storytelling selves as they seek to make sense of what is happening to them and to incorporate this new experience into their on-going life story. The different areas of importance for the person, within this life event, will be re-evaluated and have great significance for their ability to retain a sense of identity in the presence of an illness that has the potential to threaten their very existence.

If pastoral or spiritual care is to be of benefit and support it must engage at some point with that on-going inner dialogue. For this connectivity to happen there has to be a relationship of trust established that allows for sharing and exploration. There can be many inhibitions about sharing this inner dialogue and it may take time before people feel safe enough to do so. However, not knowing and understanding where the person is in relation to the effect the illness and treatment is having upon them can lead to assumptions being made and care being offered in an inappropriate way. For a minister of religion to rush to the bedside of a dying patient and administer a religious ritual without foreknowledge of the patient or the benefit of exploring what may be relevant can often alarm more than comfort all who are present. The voiceless may in fact prove not to be without a voice if we can listen to their inner voice and tune into the dialogue that may already be going on inside the person. The search for existential meaning is frequently within and our role may be as safe companions and resources for the patient, irrespective of our professional or family role.

In our present time it is frequently claimed that religion is declining and people do not need or wish for religious ministry. In the USA there has been much valuable research to demonstrate the importance of religion in health care outcomes (Koenig 1994, 1997; Pargament 1997; Pargament *et al.* 2000). However, the different cultural norms within the UK mean that the findings from these studies do not translate easily into our health care setting and culture. Current research in the UK is beginning to show that, while some people may not be overtly religious and attend places of worship, nevertheless they still participate in an existential and spiritual search for meaning and purpose in their lives (Coleman *et al.* 2002). The role of health care chaplaincy has changed a great deal from being the sole providers of traditional religious ritual to one of being a resource to people undertaking this much wider search for meaning within the illness or dying process. In 1993 the Department of Health and the main chaplaincy bodies produced an 'occupational standard' for chaplaincy, which defined the 'key purpose' as being to

> ... enable individuals and groups in a health care setting to respond to spiritual and emotional need, and to the experiences of life and death, illness and injury, in the context of a faith or belief system.
>
> (National Health Service Training Directorate 1993)

The individuals and groups referred to in this aim could be patients, families or health care staff. Historically, pastoral care has always been concerned with listening attentively to the other person and enabling them to grow and develop in their relationship with God, self and others. But there has also been at times a less comfortable prophetic voice in which chaplains and others have reflected back to the organization or society some of the issues people have shared with them in pastoral encounters. In this way the voiceless, or those not empowered to speak for themselves, may have their needs voiced in another way. Because chaplains are in, but not totally of, the organization they *can* offer an overview that can challenge any depersonalizing tendencies at various levels of interaction between those cared for, the carers and the organization (Speck 1994). In 2003 many chaplaincy departments, or spiritual care providers, would additionally see their primary aim in fairly broad terms embracing the religious *and/or* wider spiritual, existential, needs of patients, families and staff. The differentiation of spiritual from religious has been well described even though the exact nature of the non-religiously spiritual still requires further clarification (Speck 1998*a,b*). This does not mean that chaplaincy is in the process of abandoning its original religious role in order to 'capture' the wider spiritual territory. Rather what is happening is a much clearer recognition of the fact that healthy religious behaviour and practice is the outward expression of an underlying spiritual development.

Research is beginning to show (King *et al.* 1999, 2001) that many who are spiritual do not always choose to express that spirituality in a religious way and may retain a broadly spiritual stance or a philosophical approach. Whatever the underlying belief may be it leads, at critical moments in their lives, to a re-examining of the content of that belief to see whether or not it can answer the existential questions arising for the patient and family.

This can lead to a feeling of vulnerability while the belief is re-structured, re-affirmed or dispensed with as inadequate. Preliminary studies indicate that offering support to people at such times may enhance the chances of a good outcome in terms of well-being and maintenance of identity (Clarke 2001). To engage with this agenda requires the utilization of inter-personal or counselling skills to foster the safe relationship that enables mutual exploration of very personal material.

Within chaplaincy there is much experiential evidence that people find it difficult to articulate the inner struggle that they may be experiencing. This is especially so if they have previously had a religious belief but no longer follow or practise that faith. If they are presented with a religious person with whom to explore these issues then what that person represents may create barriers to effective communication and sharing. Within health care chap-laincy this has been recognized and addressed within much of the literature and training on offer and in the recruitment and use of lay (non-ordained) volunteers within a spiritual care team. Far fewer chaplains would now oper-ate in a purely religious mode but would focus on establishing a rapport with a person who is seeking to come to terms with whatever is happening to them. This is especially the case with those working within a specialist pal-liative care setting. An important part of the introduction of a chaplain to a patient either by staff or by the chaplain themselves is explaining that chap-laincy is there for all, whether religious or not. It is also important to reas-sure people that chaplaincy is not about off-loading religion onto a captive audience, nor going for the religious 'hard sell'. Respect for the person is paramount and, in the case of some illnesses where communication can be difficult, flexibility in finding ways to affirm the humanity of the other may be crucial (Stoter 1995; Wright 2002; Orchard 2001).

A research perspective

There can be misconceptions as to the willingness of patients and others to share their inner reflections and dialogue. A recent exploratory research proj-ect looked at the experience of a group of elderly spouses who had been bereaved for at least one year (Coleman et al. 2002). The study wished to dis-cover whether there was any link between the strength of a person's belief and the quality of life in old age of this group of people. Bereavement is a notoriously difficult field of research in which to recruit people and this study employed a researcher with considerable counselling experience and recruited via general practitioners (GPs). The perception by the 'gatekeepers' that this group of people were vulnerable affected ethical approval for the proposal and recruitment. The ethics committee felt it inappropriate to ask personal questions of elderly bereaved people so soon (12–24 months) after the death of the spouse. Questioning or interviewing people about their beliefs was felt by many of the 'gatekeepers' to be too intrusive. The GPs were highly selective in who they approached, selecting either those clearly well adjusted or those with difficult bereavements who might 'benefit' from the skill of the researcher/counsellor. There was a 34% agreement to join the investigation.

In the course of the investigation it became clear that the quality of the relationship between the interviewer and the participant was of great importance. However detached from the material a researcher may seek to be, one cannot ignore the dyadic relationship that is established and the effect that sharing personal, and painful, memories and experiences can have on the two people involved. Bannister *et al.* (1994) comments on the need for 'critical personal reflexivity' at several levels where the personal experiences of the researcher inform, yet do not invalidate, the findings. This is something familiar in a counselling or therapeutic encounter but often deemed inappropriate, or bad practice, in both quantitative and qualitative research. When dealing with very sensitive topics a degree of interaction is inevitable and need not be counter-productive if handled properly. Where, as in the study being described, the same people are being interviewed on several occasions some of the insights from counselling can be very helpful in maintaining sensitivity to the interviewee and to managing the 'ending' of the series of interviews. Such attributes may well be significant criteria when recruiting researchers for investigations into sensitive topics, especially where it is important to retain participant cooperation over time. This bereavement study included an exploration of the thoughts and reflections of the older people about the quality of their life, how they made sense of what had happened to them, a history of the formation and changes in their beliefs and the relevance or not of those beliefs in adjusting to the loss of their spouse. It was interesting to see that virtually all participants were able to articulate their beliefs and describe the relevance, even if some of the interviews were lengthy. It was clear that the somewhat 'over-protective' approach of the ethics committee members and the GPs was unnecessary once the relationship between the bereaved and the researcher had been established.

Because of the interactive nature of qualitative longitudinal research it became clear that there was a need for the researcher to have access to support and, when necessary, debriefing as some of the interviews revealed the presence of large areas of unresolved grief and pain. It takes a degree of altruism, courage and trust for a participant to share in this way and what

is shared must be valued. In this study the valuing was addressed by inviting the entire group to lunch at the University. In view of their advanced
age, transport was provided on a door-to-door basis and all attended, some
bringing family members as well. At the lunch the research team presented
their findings and discussed the degree of influence the findings could have
on social policy. The participants commented on the personal benefits for
them of participating in such a study, their own pleasure in thinking that
their bereavement experience was of benefit to others and their willingness
to participate in the future or to tell their friends!

Parallels for spiritual care provision

The above study has highlighted several important aspects relevant to the
provision of spiritual care. There can be different perceptions as to what is
or is not appropriate to explore with what is deemed to be a 'vulnerable'
group of people. The extent to which people are willing to share personal
material is often related to an understanding of possible benefits and a
sense that the person is genuinely interested in hearing your 'story'. In the
Schultz cartoon series *Peanuts*, one of the characters, Lucy, says 'When I
grow up I want to be a famous psychiatrist.' Charlie Brown asks 'Is that
because you are really interested in people?' 'No,' says Lucy 'I'm just nosey!'
Genuine care is, of course, not about being nosey. It is about helping the
other to explore events, past and present, for a demonstrable reason that
they can agree with.

Spiritual care, therefore, will depend on the patient and caregiver being
willing to enter together into the experience and explore without quite
knowing where it will lead. The uncertainty that this embraces can be challenging for both, but especially so for the pastoral caregiver if they have not
explored ultimate or existential issues in their own life story. One of the
reasons why health care staff find this a difficult area to engage with is that
it can quickly confront them with all the unresolved areas in their own
lives. Working with dying people already has that power and leads to the
development of a variety of defences to protect against the long-term exposure to death (Speck 1994). To explore issues concerning ultimate meaning
and purpose in another person's life is not a philosophical exercise but a
potential encounter with another person at a very deep and personal level.

Eleanor's story

Eleanor was a 43-year-old single lady when she was diagnosed as having a
malignant lump in her left breast. She was admitted to hospital for a

lumpectomy and met the chaplain during the course of a routine general visit to the ward. On admission Eleanor had not declared any religious affiliation and the first encounter with the chaplain was fairly superficial. However, the chaplain was left with a fairly clear impression of having been 'sounded out' by someone who was quite frightened at what was happening to her body and her inability to control it. She said she'd like to talk again 'but not about religion'. At the next visit Eleanor initiated a discussion about the relationship between physical illness, one's state of mind and any possible purpose behind the timing of illness. It became clear that she thought deeply about things, favoured complementary approaches and needed to explore with someone what was happening to her—but only if the other person was non-directive. Her affinity with complementary approaches to illness meant she felt somewhat trapped by finding herself dependent on 'high-tech' invasive medicine. She was pleased, however, that she had been able to exercise some control through electing for a lumpectomy rather than the recommended mastectomy. She had also agreed to a short course of radiotherapy.

The lumpectomy proceeded without problems and Eleanor managed her anxiety about the operation. Her main anxiety had related to the anaesthetic, and her inability to control what might happen to her while unconscious, rather than any fear that she might die. Radiotherapy proved to be a bigger hurdle for her. The planning and the mapping of the treatment site seemed to be all right but as the time for the first treatment got nearer, so did her anxiety until she became hysterical. She flatly refused to go to the radiotherapy department and considered 'taking my own discharge'. The ward sister called the chaplain and both spent a long time calming Eleanor; eventually she went to the department accompanied by the ward sister and chaplain who stayed with her until the treatment commenced. She completed most of the treatments but as the side-effects increased she withdrew from treatment.

During this period Eleanor had asked the chaplain to help her 'make sense of this disease' and what it was doing to her body. She did not have a close relationship with her family and saw very little of them. She did not have a partner, having split up with someone five years before her illness. She found the fact that her body was being invaded from within, by cancer, and from without by a surgeon's scalpel and radiotherapy rays, very distressing.

The inability to control what her body was doing made her very angry and this linked to a deep desire not to be dependent on anyone else. Her rather isolated life style had grown out of a desire not to depend on others because 'they can let you down as I know.' One of the reasons she was disaffected with religion was because she felt 'let down by a God who didn't protect you from hurt and pain.' Yet she also said very clearly that what she was seeking was 'inner peace' and to that end tried a wide variety of meditative techniques. In the course of a series of conversations Eleanor and the chaplain explored such words as peace, freewill, love, control, God, higher power, forgiveness, reconciliation and trust. There was a great deal of past hurt, mainly from relationships within the family and a previous lover, which created distress. She had insight into her own part in the fragmentation but struggled to know how to 'heal' the damage—some of which was also outside of her control. By listening to Eleanor and creating a safe setting where she could give voice to feelings and reactions she had not voiced before, the chaplain was able to hold the boundaries, contain her anxiety and reassure her that she could begin to put some of the pieces together and re-establish control.

The ultimate fear for many people is that the illness, the fears and the disconnectedness from others all have the power to totally annihilate the person within and I believe it is this that precipitates the existential crisis that we often see in terms of fear, anger, non-compliance and so on. Working with Eleanor in this way seemed to enable her to make some adjustment and, apart from a crisis four years later (following the collapse of a thoracic vertebra) when the disease had clearly spread, she maintained a reasonably calm and positive approach. She remained in her home, drove her car again and continued to work from home for the publishers who employed her.

A year later another crisis and clear advancement of disease re-hospitalized her. She was virtually immobile, had increased back pain and almost complete resistance to medication changes, suggested treatment and people! She refused further treatment, discharged herself to the home of a relative and expected to die soon afterwards. When she did not die her sense of helplessness and anger increased and she began imagining the various ways in which death might happen. She became irritated with her carers but also wanted not to be left alone. This made the family and professional caregivers feel increasingly helpless and desire not to visit or listen to what Eleanor might actually be saying. By working as a multi-professional team the professional caregivers were able to support each other in addressing their own inadequacy to meet Eleanor's needs. They were also able to explore a variety of approaches aimed at continuing to listen to what she was 'saying' in a variety of ways and at trying to give Eleanor a greater degree of control once again. Providing factual information about the possible ways in which she might die and what palliative care could offer also enhanced her ability to have choices. The help of the palliative care nurse and chaplain to plan her funeral, as a sacred and secular occasion with a 'green woodland' burial, also eased some anxieties around the death event. Working with the family members who had agreed to take Eleanor into their home also achieved a degree of reconciliation between Eleanor and her family in respect of *some* of the past hurt as well as her current disruptive behaviour. Over several months a combined and consistent approach by the various people involved enabled Eleanor to re-discover some of the 'inner peace' she had earlier found when eventually she died.

While the chaplain had a key role at times in enabling Eleanor to address what became an existential agenda, it was the multi-professional approach that became so vital as events moved on. The health care chaplain is not the only person who can undertake this role with a patient or family (Walter 1997, 2002). There is a sense in which spiritual care (as distinct from religious care) can be everybody's concern. However, by its very nature, chaplaincy should be a vital resource to patients, families and staff and should contain people who have at least wrestled with the issues—even if they have not obtained all the answers. Chaplaincy, therefore, becomes a key resource for such spiritual/existential explorations by patients and staff, but the actual listening, reflecting and exploration can be undertaken by anyone with the time and commitment to follow where the patient leads. However, the ability and willingness does depend to a degree on the extent to which one has for oneself faced some of these issues. At a time when there is much being written about spiritual care, it is interesting to see that many health care staff still see this as a very intrusive area to explore. Some of the problems are linguistic in trying to be clear what we mean by some of the terms and concepts, but often it is the degree of personal challenge that such conversations have for the caregiver themselves.

Ordination or appointment to a religious ministry does not automatically mean that the individual has 'it all worked out'. In fact there are many clergy who find visiting sick or dying people in hospital or at home almost impossible. Being in the presence of the sick and dying can present them with such a graphic reminder of mortality that they are unable to cope with it. Training can help, but often it is more a matter of helping the individual engage with the anxieties and fears being aroused within themselves. The research study of spirituality and bereaved people has highlighted the need for the researcher to be supported. In a similar way those providing spiritual care need to have access to appropriate support. Support might be in the form of someone to whom they can take the difficult questions, or feelings, raised by the patient. This can either be in terms of how to respond and support the patient at the next meeting, or how to work through the feelings created within the caregiver following the encounter. The development of truly multi-professional working and attendance to both our own personal agenda and the unconscious processes that are attendant upon any human interaction might enable us to move forward towards a greater readiness to hear these wider needs of patients who enter a palliative care setting.

References

Bannister P, Burman E, Parker I, Taylor M and Tindall M (1994) *Qualitative Methods in Psychology: A Research Guide*. Open University Press, Buckingham.

Clarke A-M (2001) Spirituality and well-being in elderly people undergoing elective hip and knee replacement surgery. Unpublished BSc thesis, Southampton University, UK.

Coleman P, Mills M, McKiernan F and Speck P (2002) Spiritual beliefs and quality of life: the experience of older bereaved spouses. *Quality in Ageing* 3, 20–6.

Hermans HJM (1992) Telling and retelling one's self-narrative: a contextual approach to life-span development. *Human Development* 35, 361–75.

Hermans HJM, Kempen HJC and vanLoon RJP (1992) The dialogical self: beyond individualism and rationalism. *American Psychologist* 47, 23–33.

King M, Speck P and Thomas A (1999) The effect of spiritual beliefs on outcome from illness. *Social Science and Medicine* 48, 1291–9.

King M, Speck P and Thomas A (2001) The Royal Free Interview for Spiritual and Religious Beliefs: development and validation of a self-report version. *Psychological Medicine* 31, 1015–23.

Koenig HG (1994) Religion and hope for the disabled elder. In Levin JS (ed.) *Religion in Aging and Health—Theoretical Foundations and Methodological Frontiers*, pp. 18–51. Sage, London.

Koenig HG (1997) *Is Religion Good for your Health? Effects of Religion on Mental and Physical Health*. Haworth Press, New York.

National Health Service Training Directorate (1993) *Healthcare Chaplaincy Standards*. National Health Service Training Directorate, Bristol.

Orchard H (ed.) (2001) *Spirituality in Health Care Contexts*. London, Kingsley.

Pargament KI (1997) *The Psychology of Religion and Coping: Theory, Research, Practice*. Guildford Press, New York.

Pargament KI, Koenig HG and Perez LM (2000) The many methods of religious coping: development and initial validation of the RCOPE. *Journal of Clinical Psychology* 56, 519–43.

Speck P (1994) Working with dying people—on being good enough. In Obholzer A and Roberts V. (ed.) *The Unconscious at Work: Individual and Organisational Stress in the Human Services*, pp. 94–100. Routledge, London.

Speck P (1998*a*) Spiritual issues in palliative care. In Doyle D, Hanks G and MacDonald M (ed.) *Oxford Textbook of Palliative Medicine*, pp. 805–816. Oxford University Press, Oxford.

Speck P (1998*b*) The meaning of spirituality in illness. In Cobb M and Robshaw V (ed.) *The Spiritual Challenge of Health Care*, pp. 21–34. Edinburgh, Churchill Livingstone.

Stoter D (1995) *Spiritual Aspects of Health Care*. Mosby, London.

Walter T (1997) The ideology and organization of spiritual care: three approaches. *Palliative Medicine* 11, 21–30.

Walter T (2002) Spirituality in palliative care: opportunity or burden? *Palliative Medicine* 16, 133–39.

Wright MC (2002) The essence of spiritual care: a phenomenological enquiry. *Palliative Medicine* 16, 125–32.

13

Palliative care and psychology

Christine Kalus

Introduction

Clinical psychology is something of a 'latecomer' to the field of specialist palliative care, and thus this chapter will endeavour to set out the stall of the profession, and put that in the context of the world of the users and potential users. Firstly there will be a brief explanation of how one becomes a clinical psychologist, to give the reader a sense of how our professional background may influence the way we work. This will be followed by a discussion of the meaning of 'user' as understood by the profession.

What is a clinical psychologist?

Clinical psychology is a relatively recent profession to emerge within the health care system, and initially it was predominantly sited within the field of mental health. It is only in the last 15 years that clinical psychologists have achieved greater prominence in the field of physical health (Broome 1989a; Lindsay and Powell 1994).

In the early days of the profession, the work involved the administration of psychometric tests: the intelligence test and tests for neurological dysfunction, tests that were believed to have diagnostic capabilities for severe mental illness. Thus clinical psychologists were seen as an adjunct to the medical and nursing professions. The perspective of clients, or any sense of collaborative working with them, would have been seen as an anathema by

When referring directly to the work of clinical psychologists, I will use the term client throughout because that is the term most frequently used within the profession for service users.

other health care professionals. Today, while the administration of psychometric and other tests is still an important part of many clinical psychologists' expertise, there is a much greater understanding of both the strengths and limitations of such tools. The expertise that the clinical psychologist brings is to undertake a *holistic* psychological assessment, which may take a number of sessions and include the use and interpretation of the test results within that assessment.

By the mid-1960s the development of behavioural psychology began to influence the profession and psychologists developed a role that was increasingly being seen as autonomous from that of psychiatrists and other health care professionals. Emergent behavioural treatments, such as biofeedback techniques, *in vivo* exposure to feared situations, and anxiety management were seen as viable alternatives to medication for people with clinical depression and anxiety. This trend has continued with the more recent developments of cognitive behaviour therapy (CBT) in particular and cognitive analytic therapy (CAT) being seen as effective treatments for a variety of disorders both in mental and physical health settings (Roth and Fonagay 1996; National Health Service Executive 1996). Intrinsic to this way of working is the development of a partnership between the therapist and the client, such that the client is motivated to make significant changes in their lives. While this may not always be seen as explicitly working from the 'user' perspective, the clinical psychologist would argue that it is not possible to facilitate change without having a therapeutic relationship with the client. Intrinsic to this is the need for one to have a clear and empathic understanding of the client's position, as stated by, and agreed with, the client (Gendlin 1996; Lietar 1992).

Increasingly over the past 15 years clinical and health psychologists have been recognized as having a role in the field of physical health. Within this domain, they have made a contribution to the fields of diabetes, coronary heart disease, oncology, and renal disease, amongst many others (Broome 1989*b*).

Today, clinical psychologists are trained through post-graduate doctoral courses, which combine research, clinical placements in a variety of mental health settings, and training in a range of therapeutic and communication skills. They differ from counsellors or psychotherapists, mainly because of their academic background, which fits them to work as 'scientist practitioners' (Barlow *et al.* 1984), although many undertake psychotherapy or other therapy training as part of their professional development.

This enables them to undertake service evaluation and clinical and organizational research, as well as provide a clinical service and supervision as necessary. However, because of the emphasis that the training gives to the person, both as an individual and within the context of their familial and social milieu, the work is always seen as being client or person centred. This can lead to as much conflict as cohesion when working in teams, particularly when one is trying to work with two potentially opposing views—that of the bio-medical approach and that of the psychological practitioner (British Psychological Society 2001).

What is a 'user' in clinical psychology?

There are a variety of definitions of 'user' in health care and these have been addressed elsewhere in this book. However, for the purposes of this chapter, it is important to bear in mind that the clinical psychologist will define 'user' as the person or persons who require their particular professional expertise to help resolve an organizational dilemma, personal life crisis(es) or complex clinical problems. Thus the 'user' may be the management team or individuals from an organization, the identified patient, their family or carer, the clinical team, or a supervisee in a supervision setting for individuals or groups (Manpower Planning Advisory Group 1990).

The development and influence of user groups, focusing on the perspective of the patient and their family, has been profound in the field of mental health. Well-known pressure groups include Mind, which works for and with people with severe mental health problems, The Winged Fellowship, allied to people with schizophrenia, Mencap, allied to people whose lives are touched by learning difficulties, and the Alzheimer's Disease Society, as well as many others. Each of these aims to provide advocacy, care and support for those who are not necessarily able to provide this for themselves, and to support the voices of those who can. They have provided an admirable model for others to follow.

The field of physical health also has its champions of user groups; OVACOME for women with ovarian cancer, BACUP providing general information and advice for people with cancer, Headway for people with head injury, and many others. However, with one or two exceptions, the role is often perceived as peripheral, the groups tend not to be integrally involved in service development, and users are brought in, often at the end of the planning cycle, if at all. The reasons for this are complex, but one profound influence is because the medical patriarchy still tends to dominate in service planning and development. Thus the needs of patients and families tend to be seen within a pathology/treatment context, rather than from a holistic perspective, within the context of a wider social network.

It is also important to remember that people who are recently diagnosed, perhaps with a chronic, or life-limiting, condition can feel very vulnerable and are often not in a position whereby they feel they can advocate for themselves. They want 'cure' and rely on the doctor and their team for the best treatment available. This can also put the medical team in a difficult position. If the team is not person or family centred, which can be difficult in a busy out-patient clinic, they put the doctor–patient or therapeutic relationship in jeopardy from the start, with all the attendant risks of non-compliance and poor treatment outcomes (Burton and Watson 1998). Once could argue that it is the role of the medical team to help the identi-fied patient and their family through this phase to a position of greater autonomy, to become a 'collaborator' in the journey through the disease.

Therapy versus therapeutic!

It is important to distinguish between the need for a *therapeutic relationship,* which is one that all health and social welfare staff should all aspire to achieve and which can be seen as central to good collaboration between the client and the health care providers and the need for psychological *therapy.* The latter also demands that the therapist and client have a good therapeu-tic relationship. In addition they will enter into a relationship at the core of which is the management of change. This may be at the fundamental level of self-knowing or at a behavioural level of changing the way in which the client manages difficulties such as pain control, anticipatory nausea prior to chemotherapy, needle phobias, and other feared situations that they may find themselves in as a result of the treatment. Clearly this refers to those clients who are finding managing the disease process or the treatment is having a particularly damaging effect on their or their family's ability to cope, and these are the areas that a clinical psychologist is uniquely placed to help.

The therapeutic relationship

If the user of the service is to be seen as central to service development and provision, one of the questions is how are we, as health care professionals, to achieve that? To be truly 'client centred' in Rogers' terms is to be empathic, warm and genuine, and to have an unconditional positive regard for the client (Spinelli 1997; Rogers in Kirshenbaum and Henderson 1990).

These are laudable aims, but ones that are difficult to achieve on a number of levels; to have unconditional positive regard is to truly value the client and their humanity, regardless of their personal background, idiosyncratic behaviours, ethnic origins, and value system. This may be challenging if any of these are in serious conflict with our own personal or organizational values.

In addition, busy health care professionals have to balance the needs of the individual client against the complex needs of the whole service. How does one remain truly 'client centred' when, for example, one is on a busy oncology ward and there are several people who are very ill or dying, and others who are having active treatment? When many of these people have families who are in a high state of emotional arousal and you are short staffed? Or within the hospice, where again, many people are very ill or dying, families are demanding of your time, and within the tenets of 'holistic care' you want to meet their demands, but recognize that it is not going to be possible, at least on this shift? The usual strategy is to make an emotional 'retreat' from the demands and only attend to the physical, symptom-control aspects of care. The psychologist, counsellor, social worker or chaplain can deal with the rest! These are not uncommon situations. The danger is that in not attending to the emotional and psychological 'tone' of the situation, one denies both the basic humanity of the staff who have, by and large, come into their job because they want to care, and also the needs of the client and family for that care (Samarel 1991). Clients and families have a need not just for good technical medical and nursing care, but also for a relationship in which they can put their trust, and which acknowledges the reality of the situation for them, in the context of *their* lives, that is, *a therapeutic relationship*. One could argue that this is the real meaning of 'holistic'.

There is much talk about the importance of the doctor–patient or, as it is often referred to in clinical psychology, the therapeutic relationship, in the context of factors such as compliance to treatment, client satisfaction with service provision, and longer-term use of services by families (Loscalzo and Zabora 1998; Mager and Andrykowski 2002). National Service Frameworks and Service Strategy documents make an explicit demand that health care professionals in general, and doctors in particular, improve their communication skills, and better relate with the clients and the families that they encounter (Department of Health 2000; Richards 2000). However, what does the 'therapeutic relationship' mean and how does it improve the experience of not just the service users, but the multi-professional team who provide the care? Gendlin describes the importance of the therapeutic relationship as follows.

> Interpersonal interaction is the most important therapeutic avenue. Its qualities affect all the other avenues, because they all happen *within* the interaction.
>
> (Gendlin 1996).

Rogers argues that to achieve this we need ask ourselves a number of searching questions.

◆ Can I *be* in some way which will be perceived by the other as trustworthy, dependable or consistent in some deep sense?

◆ Can I *be* expressive enough as a person that what I am will be communicated unambiguously?

◆ Can I let myself experience positive attitudes towards this other person— attitudes of warmth, caring, liking, interest, respect?

◆ Can I be strong enough as a person to be separate from the other? Can I be sturdy respecter of my own feelings, my own needs as well as his? *Am I strong enough in my own separateness that I will not be downcast by his depression, frightened by his fear, nor engulfed by his dependency?* [my italics].

◆ Can I give him the freedom to be, or do I feel that he should follow my advice, or remain somewhat dependent on me, or mold himself after me?

◆ Can I receive him as he is? Or can I only receive him conditionally, acceptant of some aspects of his feelings, and silently or openly disapproving of some other aspects?

(Rogers 1958, in Kirshenbaum and Henderson 1990)

In these contexts the authors are talking about the relationship in counselling and psychotherapy, but one could easily extrapolate the principles of what they are talking about, to those of any professional who is trying to develop a good rapport with a client. For a clinical psychologist, the key is in the notion that everything one is hoping to achieve with a client happens within the 'interaction' or relationship that one is trying to develop and maintain.

To talk of the therapeutic relationship may seem daunting for some professionals, although the reality is probably both more *simple* and more *complex* than most imagine. It is about truly *being with* the person and developing an empathic understanding of what they are trying to convey, as Rogers' tenets (above) describe. There is no magic involved. What clients and their families hope is that, despite the onset of a disease, progression through treatment, and, in some cases, getting to the stage where a person is no longer suitable for active treatment, the team will maintain their understanding of the situation and stay alongside them until their death, and with the significant others into the bereavement where appropriate. Families will often remember much about the treatments their relative had and the trauma associated with it, although these memories may fade over time. However, positive staff attitudes and an ability to care can mitigate against the worst experiences and help hold the client and family through the worst times (see Box 13.1).

Box 13.1 Case example

Sonia is a very angry and distressed young girl of 19, with malignant melanoma. She is dying in a side room of a busy oncology ward and is unable to understand why the consultant who had treated her for the past 2 years is not able to come in and see her. She frequently asks what she has done to upset him.

When asked, the doctor states that he finds it very distressing to cope with young people dying, partly because he has a family with children of the same age. As a way of protecting himself when active treatment is no longer possible, he moves on to care for those he believes he can help towards 'cure'.

He is not an uncaring or 'bad' doctor. He is simply caught up in the myth that doctors are there to treat symptoms and to 'cure'. By not acknowledging that the relationship with the client and family is fundamental to a whole range of factors in treatment, he is in danger of denying their basic humanity and human needs for care and comfort in an awful situation. He is also denying himself the possible satisfaction of helping the young girl towards a better managed and possibly more peaceful death and also enabling her and her family to better understand how the health care professions also find such situations difficult to cope with.

Perhaps the difficulty is compounded by a lack of supervision for the doctor and his team. Were he able to talk his feelings and behaviours through within a safe and structured setting he may gain a greater understanding of his motivations and also acknowledge his feelings of 'failure' in such situations. He may also find himself better equipped emotionally and practically, with support from the team, to cope with similar situations in the future.

In this case it was necessary for the clinical psychologist to offer a debriefing session for the whole team, who were clearly distressed and traumatized from the care they gave to Sonia and her family. In this they were able to reflect on what they were pleased about in the care they gave as well as have the opportunity to discuss what they would like to have done differently. As a result, they discussed how they, as a team, would want to approach similar challenges in the future.

> **Box 13.1 Case example** *(continued)*
>
> Supervision and debriefing can be perceived as punitive, or making attributions of blame, particularly in the field of health and social care. Thus the clinical psychologist was careful to ensure that the culture in which the discussion took place was one of support and challenge, which is constructivist in its approach and leads to permanent individual or structural changes to which the whole team feels able to subscribe.

It may be that for health care staff, while being aware all the time of dying and death, the level of (unconscious) death anxiety they experience causes them to distance emotionally from the client and family, as a mechanism of self-protection (Firestone 1994). While this might be an understandable reaction, one is forced to ask how helpful it is for clients and families who are looking for something in addition to the biomedical aspects of care from the team. From the perspective of clinical psychology, one could see the 'client' not as the identified patient, but rather the doctor and perhaps the wider team, who may benefit from supervision, thus taking the opportunity to look more closely at their interactions with, and reactions to, 'difficult' clients and situations.

If the health care team is not responsive to the more holistic aspects of the care, there is a possibility that the client may look to complementary approaches or seek other opinions. While this is not an intrinsically bad thing, there is the potential for conflict, for example, if the team believes that clients are in danger of harming themselves.

Alternatively, the client may choose to follow another treatment path, without informing the health care team, and this can also impede the development of a trusting and co-operative relationship. It is important to remember that the aim of a good therapeutic relationship is to develop a *constructive collaboration* between the health care team and the client and their family.

Psychological therapies

While having a good relationship with the team may have a mitigating effect for many clients in terms of mental health problems, we need to recognize that still more have significant difficulty in adjusting to their disease and changed life circumstances. These may be the people who have need of therapeutic assessment and intervention (Zabora *et al.* 2001).

Despite the methodological difficulties in collecting such data, estimates of clinical depression and anxiety seem to remain at around 30–40% of the cancer population and around 50% of those receiving palliative care

(Massie and Holland 1990; Tross and Holland 1990; Burton and Watson 1998). While many of these may be treated with some symptomatic success through drug treatments, yet more may benefit from psychological intervention, for difficulties such as anticipatory nausea, pain management, relationship difficulties, existential or death anxiety, and bereavement. (MacCormack *et al.* 2001).

We can see that the intervention with Moira (Box 13.2) illustrates that to be client centred, one needs to understand their view, as far as is possible, and help them work with what they believe to be important. There may be times when, as we could see with Moira, this was in distinct contrast to what the referring team had hoped would be the outcome—a more compliant and less disruptive 'patient'. It is also difficult to assess or define the outcome as demanded by evidence-based practice both because the issues for Moira were process issues, and also because measuring outcome from a palliative care perspective is notoriously difficult.

Box 13.2 Case example

Moira, 57, was dying from advanced metastatic breast cancer. She had had the disease for 10 years and used the experience to radically alter her life. Within 2 years of her diagnosis she left her long-term partner and a lucrative job in the City to retrain as an artist and had lived an alternative lifestyle for some years.

She was referred to the psychological services because she 'keeps turning up at out-patients angry and resentful of her lot. She will not comply with pain control regimes. Please assess her and help her see she needs to change her attitude.' When the clinical psychologist first met Moira she met a very angry and disturbed person. Moira's story is of an abused life, both as a child and in her long-term relationship, which she had left about 8 years previously. She felt the past 10 years had been the most 'freeing' of her life and she had developed a somewhat nomadic lifestyle as she strongly believed that she had an artistic and spiritual journey that needed to be completed before she died, which she knew would be fairly soon. The 'problem' she identified was that the medical team were 'outrageous' in their demands that she attended for treatment when she believed she 'needed' to be elsewhere and that they were disregarding of her wish to set up a support group in the out-patient setting. Moira felt strongly that these should incorporate staff and clients, have user feedback sessions and an active involvement in redeveloping

Box 13.2 Case example *(continued)*

the way services are provided. She also believed the staff disregarded her because of her alternative lifestyle and she spoke frequently of treatment being a re-experiencing of the abuse she hoped she had left behind some years ago.

In relation to her artistic aspirations, Moira believed that she had a project to complete and the 'hassles' she was experiencing from the medical team were impeding her progress here.

Given the nature of the referral and the medical team's frustration with Moira's behaviour, the development of a cognitive behaviour therapy programme designed to address and modify some of her automatic negative thoughts and the behavioural response to these would have been fitting. However, given Moira's explicit mistrust of and anger towards the professionals involved in her care, the clinical psychologist decided to work in an explicitly Rogerian or client-centred way, working with the issues that Moira felt were important to her, particularly given her poor prognosis. The therapy consisted of developing a trusting relationship with Moira, as she felt she had been unable to do this with other people, particularly professionals, for a number of years. Once a position was established where the clinical psychologist and Moira felt able to collaborate in her therapy, she identified and prioritized the issues that were important to her and she started to resolve them where possible.

Working through these issues allowed Moira to better understand her own motivations and some of the reasons why she became so angry and uncooperative with professionals. She began to make explicit links between some of her *present* behaviours to *past* physical and emotional abuse meted out (predominantly) by men in her private and personal life. As a result she became better able to recognize the 'triggers' for her aggression and non-compliance, and thus, in the main, modify her behaviour through the use of relaxation and positive imagery and positive self-talk to enable her to recognize the difference between her present and past relationships. One issue that she recognized she would have to 'let go' of was the out-patient group. She felt, after having talked with a number of the team in the clinic, that the time was not right for such a group. She recognized that whatever time she had left would be more productively spent concentrating on re-engaging with her children, from whom she had been estranged for some time, finishing her art project and managing the details of her death once she was admitted to the specialist unit for terminal care. She was not able to establish a trusting relationship with the

> **Box 13.2 Case example** *(continued)*
>
> hospital team, as this was not one of her priorities, although they achieved a mutual, if distanced, respect for each other and she was able to comply with at least some of the treatments they wanted her to undertake.
>
> Moira died as she had lived the past few years of her life—angry, in control and with the people she wanted around her.

There is a great deal talked about evidence-based practice in the health care system; this is a laudable aim, particularly when one is looking at the administration of expensive, toxic and potentially lethal drugs and treatments that are used in oncology and palliative care, and no less so when trying to evaluate the benefits of psychological interventions (National Health Service Executive 1996; Roth and Fonagay 1996).

When one is talking about psychological support and therapeutic interventions however, the situation becomes more difficult to analyse and the gold standard of research, the randomized control trial, should be seen as only one of the research and evaluation tools in the armoury of clinicians. One also needs to explore qualitative methods, which can be just as rigorous and often more challenging in terms of what the researcher finds out about their own way of working, as well as the research questions they may be addressing (Reason and Rowan 1998; Bromley 1986).

What do users want? Patients, families and clinicians

When we look at the needs of clients and their families, the picture becomes more confusing. The experience of living with cancer is a varied and complex one and is not static. Thus one has to be flexible and responsive to the changing needs of the client and family, from a social and psychological as well as a medical perspective. A recent American survey (Harvard Medical School of Public Affairs 2001) suggests that significant numbers of clients now make use of complementary therapies. They are driven by a number of motivations, including a wish to experience 'optimum' health, a dissatisfaction with current allopathic treatments, and when ill, a desire to return to healthy functioning and a dissatisfaction with the iatrogenic effects of many traditional treatments. One can speculate that this is also a growing trend in the UK. Centres such as the Bristol Cancer Help Centre, as well as the development of complementary health centres and spiritual healing associations and the use of the Internet to gain, albeit unregulated, information, will encourage those people who are disillusioned with traditional health provision to seek other sources of help.

Palliative care is perhaps one of the few providers of health care that is prepared to countenance some forms of complementary therapies. While many complementary therapies are still seen as 'fringe', clients frequently report the value of having relaxation therapies, reflexology and other approaches that can be seen as contributing to good self-care and positive self-esteem and offering the potential reduction in levels of stress and depression (Barraclough 1994; Yapko 1995; Milton 1998; Shapiro and Safer 2002). More recently 'mindful' approaches, based on integrating Eastern meditation with Western theoretical cognitive psychology, are being applied to the maintenance of physical and mental health and have been demonstrated to have positive effects for those who practise them (Langer 1989; Segal *et al.* 2002; Jones and Childs 2002). However, complementary therapies are still not universally offered within palliative care settings, and where they are they tend to be provided by volunteers rather than be seen as core services. This may change, as clients become more closely involved as collaborators in the provision of health care, although one must never underestimate the anxiety this can engender within the service provider. As Newnes states

> We need to open doors. Doing so requires professionals develop a 'there but for the grace of God go I' position. We act as if users of services are somehow radically different from ourselves, but of course any clinical psychologist might also have been or become a user of services. As well as involving service users in planning, management, staff interviews, training, research design and practice, we need to think about what we want from services, and would want should we find ourselves in the system. ... Much of this, of course, is about levelling out the power imbalance between professionals and service users, reducing the 'them and us' dichotomy.
>
> (Newnes 2001)

A recent survey of satisfaction with, and key events in, psychotherapy with bereaved people and people with cancer demonstrated that clients' needs were often for someone to listen non-judgementally and to allow them to express their thoughts and feelings openly and in a safe environment (Kalus 2001). The following comments represent views of the clients.

Question: Was there anything the psychologist said or did that was

(a) Helpful?

'I felt that she really listened and understood' (husband of woman with motor neurone disease (MND))

'Just having someone to talk to' (bereaved husband)

'Listening intently' (man with lung cancer)

'Everything: drawings, particularly working with my "Visions"' (young woman with breast cancer)

'Listened and prompted' (bereaved wife)

(b) unhelpful?

'... I felt she was cold and dispassionate, and showed a lack of understanding' (bereaved husband)

'I am not sure that the psychologist was the right person for me to see, and I am not sure either of us was sure why my GP had asked me to go and see her' (young man with malignant melanoma)

Question: Have you changed since you first came here?

'Yes, more positive with more self-esteem' (bereaved female client)

'More able to cope with the different stages of my cancer, and more positive too' (woman with bladder cancer, undergoing chemotherapy)

'More at ease with the situations of the past' (bereaved mother)

'Facing up to what it was like. Far more honest about my feelings' (bereaved female client)

'I have been reassured that my response to grief is "normal"' (bereaved female client)

'I have learnt that I must be kind to myself' (husband of a woman with MND)

These comments may serve to highlight the point that Newnes (2001) makes, that we need to better understand the needs of users, and also the stance taken by Smail (1996), that it may be necessary for clinical psychologists and psychotherapists to lay aside complex explanations for therapeutic change. Rather to take a more *humane* approach, which recognizes the clients' need for basic human contact and to be *truly listened* to.

Present status—future directions

The current position with regard to the involvement of clients in service development has not gone beyond being 'token' or a position of rhetoric in many instances. Professionals are anxious that their status, or perhaps more accurately, their failings are at risk. This may be particularly relevant when working with people who are dying. We know that the assessment and management of symptom control at the end of life is often difficult for the health care team and at variance from the view of patients and relatives (Higginson and McCarthy 1993). This may be in part because many health care professionals are anxious that their vulnerability may be exposed when they cannot 'cure' someone and, as in the example cited earlier, they avoid the client altogether, rather than risk such exposure.

Many of the pressure groups, including user groups, have been set up because of dissatisfaction with the care that they, or someone close to them, have received. While many do work in collaboration with the health care team, many others see themselves as having little influence, and the power of the professionals is perceived as remaining in the ascendancy. To have true collaboration, we have, as Newnes argues, to 'level out the power imbalance' (Newnes 2001).

Professionals are also naive if they believe that clients are not taking the responsibility for their care into their own hands. The recently much publicized book by Gearin-Tosh (2002) who took responsibility for the treatment of his disease is an object lesson to professionals and clients alike. He decided that he did not want conventional treatment for his myeloma and chose radical alternatives instead. He calls his book a 'medical mutiny' and has been much criticized by clients and professionals (Sunday Times Supplement 2002). However, despite this, he continues to refuse traditional treatments and chooses to undertake complementary and, to some extent, untested therapies, and he has continued to survive long after the professionals predicted he would. He may win sympathy from others who are either desperate or disillusioned enough (or both) to follow his lead.

Related to the path Gearin-Tosh followed is the emergent field of psychoneuroimmunology (PNI) defined as

> ... what happens in our minds at the level of our perception (and our emotional reaction to that perception) can have real effects on our physiology (our physical response) and more specifically, our immune systems. This is not new at all, and ancient wisdom has always encouraged us to focus on maintaining a 'healthy' mind in order to maintain a healthy body. It is only now that we are able to prove and understand the connections.
>
> (De Kooker 2002)

The means to achieve the 'wellness' and self-cure that PNI implies lie in the hands of the client themselves. This involves working on one's emotional state, through the various means of psychotherapy, altering one's lifestyle, including diet, exercise and so on, using biofeedback mechanisms to maintain good levels of relaxation, as well as many other therapies that could be seen as 'fringe'. It is also important to bear in mind that although many of these therapies do not necessarily have a sound evidence base now, this does not mean that in years to come, when our research methods have become sufficiently refined such that they are able to assess these more subtle methods of (potential) change, we will not be able to evaluate them in their own right. This is an area where psychologists are well equipped to help with both the science and the practice of many of these therapies.

Much of this information is available on the Internet, as well as in the press and magazines. It is possible to speculate that as the current cohort of people who grew up in the 1950s and 1960s ages, they are the generation who will increasingly want alternative treatments and will have the articulacy and education to demand they are available as part of the health care system. If the approaches are seen as helpful, the trend will be passed on through the generations.

This approach is not without its critics: academic, individual and societal. Much of the debate centres on the methods and assumptions that are made in the name of PNI. A major difficulty for many is that because the approaches are not necessarily 'mainstream', it is difficult to find suitable practitioners and one often has to pay for treatments. Additionally, professional regulation of many practitioners is patchy and the client needs to be selective in how they choose. Despite this, there is no doubting the commitment of those involved in the research, nor the impressive work coming from many of the research centres (Pert 1997; Hirschberg and Barasch 1995; Kiecolt-Glaser and Glaser 1994; NHS Research Support Unit 2000).

If all of this is to make sense, then we need to incorporate clients and families in every facet of the health care process. This is going to be a huge challenge for health care providers and clients and families alike, because it demands a demystification of the techniques used by professionals and a willingness from the clients and families to participate as equals, rather than in a passive way.

From the perspective of clinical psychology, this will involve a culture shift from hiding behind the mystique of being a 'blank screen' onto which the client can project their innermost thoughts and feelings, to finding ways in which they can learn to change unhelpful behaviours. We need to find ways to maintain appropriate and helpful boundaries and at the same time work on reducing the (often unhelpful) mystique that comes with the label 'clinical psychologist'.

Jane Wardle, a clinical psychologist who has worked for many years as a researcher in the psychological effects of cancer, was diagnosed with chronic lymphocytic leukaemia (CLL) 3 years ago. In a recent article about her experience she writes

> In the medical community it is a time of extraordinary change in attitudes. The concept of the 'expert patient' is sweeping through the NHS and fast replacing the concept of 'patient as victim'. Part of this comes from the seismic effect of the internet, making information that was once restricted to doctors and scientists almost equally available to patients ... and although it won't always be easy, I hope we are in a new era where patients and doctors will work together to understand and treat disease and people with a foot in both camps might be able to make a special contribution.
>
> (Wardle 2002)

To develop the right culture, staff are going to have to develop a greater willingness to look at their current practice, not from the perspective of blame, but more from one of reflective practice. This can be achieved in a number of ways, but as the client and professional have to develop a sound therapeutic relationship, so must professionals between each other. The challenge of working together from a perspective of nurture and honesty, when the health care culture has fostered the opposite for many years, is not to be underestimated. One way to achieve this is to develop joint supervision and training for professionals and clients alike. Another is perhaps to listen more closely to our clients and their families and to find out how *they* survive and develop in what often seems a hostile and unforgiving world. We have a lot to learn.

References

Barlow DH, Hayes S and Nelson RO (1984). *The Scientist Practitioner. Research and Accountability in Clinical and Educational Settings.* Pergamon Press, Oxford.

Barraclough J (1994). *Cancer and Emotion. A Practical Guide to Psychooncology.* Second edition. Wiley, Chichester.

British Psychological Society (2001). *Working in Teams.* BPS Publications, Leicester, UK.

Broome AK (ed.) (1989a). *Health Psychology. Processes and applications.* Llewlyn SP. Chapter 7. *Caring: The costs to nurses and relatives.* pp. 114–131. Chapman and Hall, London.

Broome AK (ed.) (1989b). *Health Psychology. Processes and applications.* Robinson EJ. Chapter 8. *Patients' contributions to the consultation.* pp. 131–153. Chapman and Hall, London.

Burton M and Watson M (1998). *Counselling People with Cancer.* Wiley, Chichester.

De Kooker M (2002). *Psychoneuroimmunology. An overview.* The wellness support programme. www.wellness.org.za.

Department of Health (2000). The NHS Cancer Plan. Department of Health, Leeds.

Firestone RW (1994). Psychological defenses against death anxiety. In: Neimeyer R (ed.) *The Death Anxiety Handbook.* Taylor and Francis, London.

Gearin-Tosh M (2002). *Living Proof. A Medical Mutiny.* Scribner, London.

Gendlin ET (1996). *Focussing Oriented Psychotherapy. A Manual of the Experiential Method.* Guildford Press, New York.

Harvard Medical School of Public Affairs (2001). Study indicates alternative medicine is here to stay. www.hms.harvard.edu.

Higginson I and McCarthy M (1993). Validity of the support team assessment schedules. Do staffs' ratings reflect those made by patients and their families? *Palliative Medicine* 7:219–28.

Hirschberg C and Barasch MI (1995). *Remarkable Recovery. What Extraordinary Healings Can Teach Us About Getting Well and Staying Well.* Headline, London.

Jones A and Childs D (2002). Mindfulness. *Clinical Psychology* 11:23–7.

Kalus C (2001). Satisfaction with clinical psychology service in specialist palliative care. Unpublished report, Portsmouth Healthcare Trust.

Kiecolt-Glaser JK and Glaser R (ed.) (1994). *Handbook of Human Stress and Immunity.* Academic Press, New York.

Kirshebaum H and Henderson VL (ed.) (1990). *The Carl Rogers Reader.* Constable, London.

Langer EJ (1989). *Mindfulness: Choice and Control in Everyday Life.* Harvill, London.

Lietar G (1992). *Psychotherapy Process Research. Paradigmatic and Narrative Approaches. Helping and Hindering Processes in Client Centred/Experiential Psychotherapy: A Content Analysis of Client and Therapist Post-session Perceptions.* Sage, London.

Lindsay SJE and Powell GE (1994). *The Handbook of Clinical Adult Psychology.* Second edition. Routledge, London.

Loscalzo MJ and Zabora JR (1998). Care of the cancer patient: response of family and staff. In: Bruera E and Portenoy RK (ed.) *Topics in Palliative Care. Volume 2.* Oxford University Press, Oxford.

MacCormack T, Simonian J, Lim J *et al.* (2001). 'Someone who cares': A qualitative investigation of cancer patients experience of psychotherapy. *Psycho-oncology* 10:52–66.

Mager WM and Andrykowski MA (2002). Communication in the cancer "bad news" consultation: patient perception and psychological adustment. *Psycho-Oncology* 11:35–47.

Manpower Planning Advisory Group (1990). *Clinical Psychology Report.* Department of Health, London.

Massie MJ and Holland JC (1990). Overview of Normal Reactions and Prevalence of Psychiatric Disorders. In: Holland JC and Rowland JH (ed.) *Handbook of Psychooncology*. Oxford University Press, Oxford.

Milton D (1998). Alternative and complementary therapies: integration into cancer care. *AAOHN Journal* 46:454–63.

National Health Service Executive (1996). *Good Practice. NHS Psychotherapy Services in England. Review of Strategic Policy*. Stationery Office, London.

National Health Service Research Support Unit (2000). *Involving consumers in research and development in the NHS: briefing notes for researchers*.

Newnes C (2001). Clinical psychology, user involvement and advocacy. *Clinical Psychology Forum* 150:18–23.

Pert C (1997). *Molecules of Emotion*. Simon and Schuster, Sydney.

Reason P and Rowan J (ed.) (1998). *Human Inquiry in Action*. Sage, London.

Richards M (2000). Development of a supportive care strategy. Unpublished keynote address to the Seventeenth Annual Conference of the British Psychosocial Oncology Society, Leicester, UK.

Roth A and Fonagay P (1996). *What Works for Whom? A Critical Review of Psychotherapy Research*. Guildford Press, London.

Samarel N (1991). *Caring for Life and Death*. Taylor & Francis, London.

Segal ZV, Williams JMG and Teasdale JD (2002). *Mindfulness-based Cognitive Therapy for Depression. A New Approach for Preventing Relapse*. Guildford Press, New York.

Shapiro DA and Safer M (2002). Integrating complementary therapies into a traditional oncology practice. *Oncology Issues* January/February: 35–9.

Smail D (1996). *How to Survive without Psychotherapy*. Constable, London.

Spinelli E (1997). *Tales of Un-knowing. Therapeutic Encounters from an Existential Perspective*. Duckworth, London.

Sunday Times Supplement (2002). 20/27 January.

Tross S and Holland JC (1990). Psychological sequelae in cancer survivors. In: Holland JC and Rowland JH (ed.) *Handbook of Psychooncology*. Oxford University Press, Oxford.

Wardle J (2002). Physician heal thyself. *Observer Review*, 17 March.

Yapko MD (1995). *Essentials of Hypnosis*. Bruner Mazel, New York.

Zabora J, Brintzenhofeszoc K, Curbow B, Hooker C and Piantadosi S (2001). The prevalence of psychological distress by cancer site. *Psycho-oncology* 10:19–28.

14

Conclusions

Alwyn Lishman

Introduction

The common thread uniting the chapters of this book is a deep humanity, focused on improving the lot of the terminally ill. But humanity alone is rarely enough to launch endeavours or achieve substantial change. It must be coupled with drive, ingenuity and a considerable amount of know-how.

Thus we see on reading these chapters that palliative care needs to operate within complex structures—organizational, and in the broad sense, political. Alliances must be constructed between diverse groups of people and financial limitations must be faced. All of these matters require professional expertise in addition to humanitarian concern.

Such issues are well illustrated here and provided for me a much-needed educative experience. It is all too easy to take the existing status quo for granted and to overlook the struggles that have brought it into being. Yet without a keen appreciation of the context within which palliative care must operate future progress and development may be limited. Continuing advocacy is required to see that systems do not become rigid and stale, or even begin to atrophy.

We can be reassured from this compilation of papers that there is little risk that such a fate could lie ahead for palliative care. The required expertise abounds. And it is immensely encouraging to see that the 'user's voice' is widely welcomed in seeking to refine the way forward.

Personal experience

Before I found that myself and my wife were users (how I dislike the term!)— she the patient, I the carer—I had given little thought to the pathways we were destined to follow. I knew about the range of medical services we would encounter—neurological, surgical, oncological and perhaps ulti-mately hospice care—but little about the way they were linked together. Nor did I foresee the extent of support we would receive along the way. Without doubt was the latter which made the journey bearable.

To begin with we were unusually fortunate in our general practitioner, who held things together in the earlier stages and remained near the fore-front of the picture throughout. Coordination was certainly required—at one time we were attending six hospitals together!

Hospital care was often excellent, sometimes not so good. Hardest to bear for Marjorie, I think, was a drowning sense of loss of her identity as we trundled too and fro encountering an increasing number of faces. Her dearest wish at times was to be seen as she was—an individual with a life history of her own. In those hospitals with specialized nurses who came to know her well this distress was greatly lessened.

I had looked ahead with concern to Marjorie's reaction when the time came for transition from active treatment to palliative care, but in the event it was managed seamlessly. There was a good deal of overlap between the two, with both sets of medical personnel working in concert with one another for a while. Moreover the hospice staff became well known to us long before the transition occurred, thanks to the foresight of our social worker and hospice home care nurse. Attendance at a cheerful hospice day centre began while active treatment was in progress; and when the hospice took over Marjorie's care, the provision of active physiotherapy, with rewarding gains, did much to obscure the divide between hospital and hospice.

More important than this, however, were the qualities and attitudes we encountered among the hospice personnel—nurses, doctors and volun-teers. What I think we valued most were the kindness and cheerfulness of all concerned and their appreciation at all times of the uniqueness of the individual. We now encountered support from those who were comfort-able with the issues surrounding deeply threatening illness. The absence of fear and anxiety in those around was a powerful factor in reducing our own.

But perhaps I should have stressed first and foremost the value of proper communication. Hopes fulfilled and dashed—these are ultimately bearable provided all concerned are honest and straightforward. Marjorie's home care nurse and my social worker kept us informed and guided our think-ing throughout in a sensitive and talented manner. We did not feel 'on our own' as we confronted the most difficult period of our lives.

The user's voice

As it happened Marjorie survived 9 years, when the initial prognosis had tended to be gloomy; 9 years of happiness and re-affirmation and of guided preparation for the ultimate outcome. In all of this we were greatly blessed.

But what of the others less fortunate than we were? Here the user's voice has a special part to play. Perhaps no other element, on its own, can ensure so firmly that services develop in a truly person-centred fashion. This is why I have ventured to outline our personal experiences in some detail.

The users of services are at once well motivated to help and uniquely informed about areas where change is needed. But in my view it is imperative that we seek to obtain the views of those who have been less privileged and less than fully supported during their illnesses. Only in this way shall we clearly define where change is required.

General practitioners are sometimes too busy or ill-equipped themselves to provide much-needed assistance. Hospice care is even now relatively scarce in some areas of the country. For a service to be really person centred and patient focused we require as a minimum adequate numbers of personnel, and care in their recruitment and training to ensure that they are suited to the task.

Individual patients vary greatly in their reactions to the approach of the end of their lives and care must be tailored to their individual needs. This is a tall order. The training of staff who work in palliative care can scarcely be expected to encompass a full range of psychological expertise, but fortunately qualities of perceptiveness and intuition are seemingly built in to many who are attracted to work in the field. The availability in centres of excellence of a wide range of people from diverse professional backgrounds ensures, one hopes, that serious gaps will be filled. We must aim to cater, moreover for the diverse cultural needs of our clients, and here, too, only the user's voice can hope to point the way forward with accuracy.

Palliative care at the end of life is now a respected and well-established part of modern society. It reaches out for guidance towards further evolution and improvement. The users of the services currently provided will, it is hoped, be able to play a constructive role in helping to shape its future.

15

Conclusion: thoughts of a palliative care user

Fiona Broughton

I feel privileged to be asked to make a contribution to this wide-ranging and thought-provoking book. It has given me the chance to express my own thoughts about, and support for, the greater involvement of patients in the highly sensitive arena of palliative care. My view is of course one of many; personal and 'non-binding' on any other user! What is important or relevant to me, with my background, sex, wishes and aspirations may be very different to what might be important or relevant to another user.

My journey to take on the role of a palliative care user began over a year before diagnosis, with a number of visits to my family doctor with strange pains and discomfort in my shoulder, neck, and side of the chest and right arm. Then came the day when, instead of the expected acupuncture session, I heard the news that a tumour had been discovered under my collar bone. Unusual apparently. Devastating actually. What to do now? I was exceptionally fortunate in having a medical consultant in the family, who was able to draw on the knowledge and expertise of colleagues to identify where I was most likely to find the specialists who might be able to help.

The next few months followed what is no doubt a familiar pattern to the professional: scans and tests galore; a major operation, recently developed, which left me without part of my collar bone, part of a few ribs and half a lung, plus a number of other minor problems; four weeks in hospital; recalcitrant pain; and two months rest and recuperation. I was supported by my long-suffering sister and that same consultant, along with an understanding district nurse. Six weeks of intensive radiotherapy followed—and home at last!

My family doctor helped, arranged for physiotherapy support and put me in contact with a Macmillan nurse who later suggested a programme for 'younger' cancer sufferers run by my local day hospice. From that grew my interest in palliative care and in the concept of 'user involvement'.

The transition from independence—a moderately successful career in the personnel field and in business consultancy, with considerable responsibility, working long hours and coping with the usual stresses, along with community involvement as a magistrate—to that of disabled cancer patient, was difficult. I found myself in a situation where I did not know if I would survive or for how long. I was tearful and depressed, my self-confidence had vanished, as had my income. I felt lost, of no value, making no contribution to society. I was in a great deal of pain. That was 7 years ago. Thanks to the help, support and encouragement of many involved in palliative care I feel I have moved on to carve out a new life.

One aspect that has played a part in that process has been my involvement as a 'service user'. On reflection I perceive several stages. In the days and months following surgery my involvement was primarily concerned with me—asking for information and advice and for help in coming to terms with fears and worries, planning finances and adapting my lifestyle. After a while, alongside my own concerns, I recall talking and listening to others, encouraging them to talk and on occasions acting informally as an advocate. Then followed opportunities to participate in far wider arenas: contributing to the thinking, planning, organization and conduct of a conference concerned with user involvement, participating in an advisory group on a research project in this field and assessing user involvement projects and development work for recognition and awards—these examples give some idea.

As Neil Small mentions in Chapter 2, the original hospice movement was a response to the recognition of the need to better care for people 'at the most painful, critical, heart breaking time of their lives'. It can be a time when a person is unable to, or finds great difficulty in, voicing their needs and concerns, so enormous efforts to ensure these are discovered, acknowledged, respected and met whenever possible, may be required from all those involved in caring.

How this can be done will vary enormously. Determined but sensitive attempts to solicit those needs, to discover concerns (which may not yet be conscious thoughts on the part of the user) are warranted. Carers, from medical specialists to hospice volunteers, from physiotherapists and art therapists to friends and relatives, need to recognize opportunities to prompt thoughts, to watch for clues, to pose alternatives and to raise potential issues.

Many users will not be voiceless, some may even be vociferous! However, whilst some needs may be disclosed openly, others may tend to be subdued, suborned, hidden or referred to indirectly. I am no psychiatrist so the question of why I will leave to others. I only know, from my own journey, that all of these factors have played a part in my attempts to express wants and worries, hopes and desires. So do, please, watch for all these subterfuges! Vehicles such as informal discussion groups, on any subject, may disclose some need; one-to-one conversations others; comments from one user to another are often a good source—I am not talking about eavesdropping but people deliberately ensure a conversation will be overheard. Some subjects may be extremely difficult for an individual to raise and such an indirect method can make it possible. It is often easier to express worries to a fellow sufferer than to a carer, however sympathetic. Perhaps a key point to remember is that what may be everyday matter-of-fact problems to a professional can be devastatingly embarrassing or delicate especially to a newly diagnosed patient.

What other techniques can be used, on an individual level? Technology has advanced so rapidly that I would hope e-mails, on-line chat rooms and similar tools can and are being added to earlier methods such as suggestion boxes, ansaphones or focus groups.

For the individual, concerned and involved in their own care and personal issues, participation and involvement can, and I believe should, move on and develop further. Citizen participation in a multitude of fields is being increasingly valued and recognized as beneficial in many ways and thus encouraged—not merely as something 'politically correct'. Whilst there may be particular difficulties in finding ways in which seriously or terminally ill palliative care users can be involved, these are not insurmountable. Some may be longer term and formalized, others could be 'one-offs' and informal.

Why then does not every hospice and organization, charity, research body and health service management group with a role in the management and development of palliative care have, as a minimum, at least one user, with the same voting powers, authority and responsibility as other members, as a matter of course? I see that step forward, from user involvement in their own care, to a recognition and desire to encourage and enable users to take on a far wider role in the management, organization, planning and development of palliative care services, as the current challenge for all bodies in the sector. Backing from the present government is invaluable but a real commitment is needed by all parties, not merely 'going through the motions', taking the easiest route or limiting involvement by limiting full participation. User involvement is for me translating users' experience into better services.

Although people may change, a person with cancer, motor neurone disease, HIV/AIDS or heart disease does not suddenly lose all their knowledge, skills, education or intellect or their ability to debate, learn, manage, plan, organize, evaluate, make decisions or balance options, even budget! Professionals do not invariably know what is best for a patient needing palliative care. It may be demanding, even threatening, to allow those receiving your care to play a more substantial role but it could be of great benefit; you might even grow to like it!

Index